Health in the New Testament

By Dr. Chase Faldmo, D.C.

Dr. Chase Faldmo, DC

Health in the New Testament

Published by Chase Faldmo, D.C.

ISBN: 978-2-2971-4449-0

Healingplaybook.com

DISCLAIMER:

"Healing Playbook: Non-invasive detox secrets to save time, money, and resources" is a book (hereinafter specifically referred to as "the book") containing a study of a form of unorthodox and alternative system of diagnosis of illness in theory. "Healing Playbook, LLC" shall mean and include the book, its owners, authors, publishers contributors and its website "www.healingplaybook.com" (hereinafter called and referred to as "Healing Playbook"). "Client" means and includes any person who uses the services or participates in activities arranged and conducted by Healing Playbook, LLC and the readers and purchasers of the book including their agents and representatives. All that contained herein shall be severable and be given force of law regardless of any part rendered invalid, defective or void by operation of law or any other reason.

All that stated hereunder shall be binding on all purchases/contracts of services and shall be part and parcel of the same and the client agrees and confirms that:

1. All descriptions, illustrations, examples provided in the book shall only be for informing the procedures, methods, materials used in the book and the book is to be used only for educational purposes.

2. No warranty is given of the effects of the procedures or methods used. Each person shall experience these effects individually distinct to that of the effects experienced by another.

3. There shall be no warranty for the intensity or mildness experienced of the effect of the procedures and methods used. The intensity or mildness may vary due to the unique condition of the client's physique and the mind.

4. Any mental or physical discomfort caused shall not be intentional as all information provided by the book are to make a person, comfortable, vitalized and free from a particular illness. The client hereby agrees that the client shall immediately remove himself/herself from any situation which cause or may cause discomfort. The client further agrees not to hold Healing Playbook, LLC liable for such discomfort or hurt experienced.

5. Healing Playbook shall not be liable for Injury or loss arising due to the client not immediately removing himself /herself from such situation which cause discomfort, injury or loss.

6. Pro-longed exposure to discomfort which is not conveyed to Healing Playbook, LLC shall absolve Healing Playbook, LLC of liability of injury, loss emanating from such exposure.

7. Instances mentioned in Clauses 2,3,4 may rarely occur as all procedures and methods used are closely monitored and controlled.

8. Any injury, loss, discomfort experienced by the client due to client's negligence, recklessness, inaction, failure to follow instructions shall be borne by the client himself/herself and shall not hold Healing Playbook, LLC liable.

9. Any loss caused by accident shall lie where it falls. Client suffering loss shall not hold Healing Playbook, LLC liable for such loss.

10. The client understands and may agree to undergo/be part of the activities provided in the book on his/her own volition, knowing the outcomes of such activity. Wherefore, the client forfeits the right to initiate legal action against Healing Playbook, LLC anything contrary to what is agreed hereunder.

11. The client understands, agrees and approves that the information provided in the book is not in anyway approved by a Food and Drug Administration (FDA) or any other government institution, but based on a personal study.

12. The Client agrees to seek the assistance and advise of a medical healthcare professional who is competent, approved by the government and permitted to give such service before participating in any of the activities mentioned in the book and follow up only if the healthcare professional approves or declares the information provided in the book to be harmless.

13. Activities/elements and their doses stated in the book are offered without any express or implied warranty, including, but not limited to, the implied warranties of merchantability and fitness for a particular purpose and are disclaimed in each case. In no event shall Healing Playbook, LLC be liable for any direct, indirect, incidental, special, exemplary, or consequential damages (including, but not limited to, procurement of substitute goods or services; loss of use or profits; personal injury or business interruption, physical or mental hurt or discomfort) however caused and on any theory of liability, whether in contract, strict liability,

or tort (including negligence or otherwise) arising in anyway, even if advised of the possibility of such damage.

Healing Playbook, LLC

SPECIAL THANKS:

To my wonderful and beautiful wife, Ashley, and to my kids who I love so much, Reagan, Amanda, Collins, and Ox. Thank you for your patience and sacrifice. I promise this will all pay off in the end.

Table of Contents

INTRODUCTION

This book should have been my first. When I was sixteen years old, I was a thriving, healthy athlete until I underwent hydrocele surgery. After the surgery, I took painkillers and anti-inflammatories, which caused large ulcers to develop in my stomach. In an attempt to address this, I was prescribed even more medications. To make a long story short, I lost fifty pounds, my organs began to shut down, and despite consulting some of the best doctors across the country, none of them could help me. I underwent every lab test and diagnostic procedure available, yet they could not determine the cause of my illness or how to help me recover. After almost two years, I found myself near the end.

In 2008, by the grace of God, I discovered the principles of frequencies, physics, voltage, and nutrition. I applied these principles to my own body and began to notice improvements in my health within just two weeks. After a year, I felt better than before I had gotten sick, after struggling and nearly dying for two years.

Through this experience, I realized the importance of the body. When my body was unwell, I also felt it affected me spiritually. We need both our spirit and body; together, they make up our soul.

I received countless prayers and blessings during my illness, and I truly believe I wouldn't have made it through without them. When it comes to healing the body, the spiritual aspect is essential. I have often seen that prayers and spiritual support play a crucial role in recovering from chronic illnesses or conditions.

In my experience, I also realized that I needed physical tools to help me heal. God works through faith and works. We must have faith to heal, but we also need to put forth the effort. Part of what I will share in this book will incorporate faith and action, which is why this should have been the first book I wrote.

For the body to heal, I like to compare it to a plant. In nature, plants can survive, thrive, and produce offspring. Similarly, as humans, we not only want to survive, but we also want to thrive, replenish, and renew ourselves. Additionally, we aspire to have children and give them the happiest, healthiest lives possible, much like how plants strive to produce seeds that not only survive but also thrive.

Some people cannot have children, but when we think about the term "offspring," it's important to consider that it can mean more than just having kids. It can also refer to making the world a better place and leaving a lasting legacy. Many incredible individuals I know were unable to have children, yet the legacies they created and their nurturing qualities positively impacted so many lives.

It is human nature to desire to thrive in any situation, just like plants. For this to happen, we need to maintain our health. Let's examine how plants stay healthy. The first essential requirement for plants is sunlight. Similarly, we also need sunlight, as it helps to correct something called polarity.

The body is like a rechargeable battery. If the power in our body drops to zero, then the polarity flips. It is like putting a rechargeable battery upside down in a battery charger; it will not hold a charge. Luckily, there are several ways to correct polarity.

First is light from the sun. The sun produces a beneficial type of energy known as scalar frequencies, which correct polarity. Other things I have seen that correct polarity include prayer, meditation, and essential oils. You can mechanically reproduce scalar frequencies.

For a plant to survive, it requires electromagnetic frequencies. When plants are rooted in the ground, they draw power from the soil, which helps them thrive. We can experience a similar phenomenon. By walking barefoot on grass, dirt, sand or by exercising, we can generate energy in our bodies. Since our muscles are piezoelectric, this activity enables our bodies to recharge fully.

Life on Earth depends on lightning, which transfers energy to the ground. This is why grounding is so beneficial: it enhances the frequency and vibration within our bodies.

We also receive frequencies in our bodies through sound. Plants absorb sound, vibration, and frequency from various sources, including bees. However, it's not just bees; butterflies and other insects, as well as birds, play a role too. These creatures visit the openings of flowers, which helps generate frequency and elevate the vibration of the plants, enabling them to thrive.

Sound has the same effect on people, which is why I created a membership with healing sound frequencies that align with the patterns God created in nature. My goal is to help people raise their frequency and vibration for healing.

Lastly, you'll notice that plants constantly strive to grow upward, despite facing challenges from wind, temperature, and various other factors. Similarly, we as individuals need movement, exercise, and proper posture to thrive, yet these fundamental principles have been overlooked in our culture.
But we are starting to return to these principles. We will be stronger and happier as we return to the principles that our ancestors knew and practiced.

As I have read and studied the scriptures, I have realized that the greatest Healer of all time is our Savior, Jesus Christ. He is the Healer of all things, and I will share many of these principles in this book. He used both faith and works to heal people. That's the powerful principle I want you to learn. Additionally, I want to emphasize the importance of scripture in teaching you valuable insights relevant to your field of expertise.

After I recovered from my sickness, I was blessed to meet my beautiful wife, Ashley. Together, we've had multiple children, and I graduated as a Doctor of Chiropractic.

Throughout my career, I have seen thousands of patients from around the world with some of the most unique conditions. Many people often ask me where I learned about frequency, physics, nerves, and various health techniques. The most significant source of my knowledge comes from the scriptures. Again, Christ does all the healing, but I will share the principles and insights I have learned, serving as tools and instruments in His hands to help many people heal.

CHAPTER 1: ELISABETH AND ZACHARIAS

In Luke 1:1, we read about a woman named Elisabeth and a man named Zacharias, who were older and at an age when they could not bear children (King James Version). In Luke 1:8-9, we read that Zacharia's duty was to burn incense at the temple's altars (KJV).

Now, this is an essential key point. When we serve God, He will always reward us and call us to do specific callings to help our spirit and body learn and grow. So Zacharias was called to burn incense for a reason.

The first cranial nerve, the olfactory nerve, comes from the brainstem and helps with your sense of smell. Smell activates the midline of your brain so your left and right brain can communicate. The midline of the brain is also associated with the bladder power line. The bladder is one of the most influential power lines in the body.

So Zacharias, just by burning incense, activated this system. Not only that, but certain parts of the brain fire during intimacy, and one of them for men is the ventral lateral thalamus. And the ventral lateral thalamus is influenced by smell.

So, just by smelling, Zacharias could activate these nerves and power systems, allowing him to become more fertile.

I have also seen this phenomenon in our day. Since 2019, many people have lost their smell after being sick. Along with this side effect, I began noticing that they not only had less desire to be intimate, but they were also less fertile.

Once you restore your sense of smell, it is incredible how much the power line of intimacy is influenced, not to mention fertility. But it can't just be any smell. Zacharias had access to more natural scents in his day. Unfortunately, in our day, there are so many artificial scents and aromas that have thrown off our true sense of smell. When people try to restore it artificially, the body rejects it. But using more natural smells, such as essential oils, provides your body the power and frequencies it needs to thrive.

Not only was he benefiting from the incense, but the very presence in the temple also elevated his frequency and vibration. Temples are constructed with specific materials such as stone, rocks, crystals, and granite, all of which possess higher frequencies. Additionally, they incorporate specific geometric patterns that allow scalar frequencies from the sun to be absorbed within them. As a result, everyone inside and around the temple benefits from this energy.

Temples utilize the principles of Platonic solids, thereby raising the vibration of everyone inside.

In Luke 1:11-13, we read about an angel appearing to Zacharias at the right side of the altar of incense (KJV). This detail suggests that God pays attention to the specifics in our lives, as the angel's placement was intentional. We can draw two significant principles from this encounter. The first principle relates to cranial nerve two, also known as the optic nerve, which is responsible for vision. When the angel appeared to Zacharias' right, it activated the optic nerve tract, stimulating more activity in the left side of the brain.

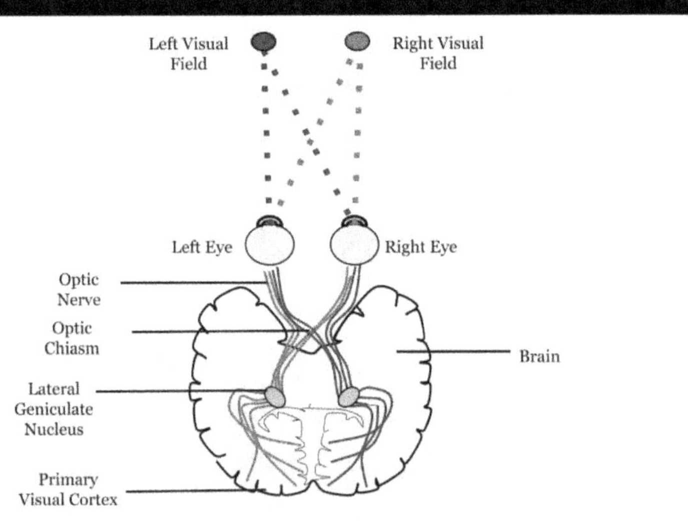

Image: "Neural pathway diagram" by Mads00 is licensed under CC BY 4.0

Now, the left side of the brain has more masculine polarity, and when you raise the power of the left side of the brain, it activates testosterone, which also makes Zacharias more fertile.

When the angel appeared, it activated several nerves, including cranial nerve three, which is quite significant. Many people describe the bright light associated with angelic encounters, and this light causes the eyes to react by constricting the pupils. Cranial nerve three plays a crucial role in this process, as it is responsible for pupil constriction. This nerve is part of the parasympathetic nervous system, which helps the body rest and digest, but it is also essential for arousal.

The angel also told Zacharias not to be afraid when he appeared to him. I will dive deeper into this topic in a later chapter, particularly regarding Mary, but it's important to emphasize that Zacharias activated several nerves that contributed to his fertility, including the olfactory nerve, which is stimulated by smell. The key point is that he was serving God in the temple. By being in that sacred space, God blessed him, placing him in the right situation at the right time to enhance his fertility.

This relates to cranial nerve one, but also to the angel's appearance, which brought light and activated two additional nerves. This activation stimulated the left side of his brain, increasing testosterone levels and thus enhancing his fertility. This is why the angel promised him he would have a son, who was to be named John.

If our nerves and our body's power lines are stronger, we will be more fertile, which I have observed in patients.

CHAPTER 2: ALCOHOL

In Luke 1:15, the angel describes John the Baptist, stating he will "be great in the sight of the Lord and shall drink neither wine nor strong drink (KJV)." This indicates that John the Baptist will abstain from alcohol, highlighting an important health biohack that many people overlook today. Additionally, Ephesians 5:18 says to "be not drunk with wine…but be filled with the Spirit (KJV)."

Alcohol consumption leads to dysbiosis, which disrupts the balance of bacteria in the gut and ultimately causes a leaky gut. A leaky gut allows harmful substances to pass into the body, compromising our defense against toxins.

Additionally, research shows that alcohol can interfere with the absorption of essential nutrients, including glucose, glutamine, vitamins B1, B2, B9, C, iron, zinc, and selenium (Butts et al., 2023). These nutrients are vital for various bodily functions, so let's first focus on glucose.

Glucose is well-known for its importance in neurology; our nerves require glucose, oxygen, and energy to function effectively. I believe that when nerves are unable to properly utilize glucose, it can lead to a range of neurological disorders, making it a vital nutrient.

Vitamin C is also necessary for the immune system to function correctly (Carr & Maggini, 2017). Vitamin B1 and zinc are of special interest to me as well. Vitamin B1 and zinc help your body to produce stomach acid to help digest your food.

I notice daily that many patients have undigested proteins. This is because when we eat our food, our body is in protein form, and stomach acid helps break it down. When we break down the proteins properly into amino acids, that's what our body can digest and absorb. However, undigested proteins are a huge problem today.

Lastly, selenium is needed for the thyroid to function (Zuo et al., 2021). So when you can absorb selenium and your thyroid is not working correctly, that controls the ATP in your body, giving you significantly decreased energy. When you think about all these minerals that are not absorbed because of alcohol, you can describe many of the chronic diseases and illnesses that occur in our day due to alcohol consumption.

John the Baptist's ability to avoid alcohol contributed significantly to his greatness as a leader.

CHAPTER 3: THE EIGHTH DAY, SPEAKING YOUR VOICE AND THE LUNG/LARGE INTESTINE

Let's revisit Zacharias, the father of John the Baptist. Before John the Baptist was born, an angel appeared to Zacharias. In Luke 1:18-20, we read that Zacharias did not believe the angel's message. As a result, the angel made him dumb or unable to speak (KJV).

We later learn that the baby was born and it says in Luke 1:59 that on the eighth day they came to circumcise the child (KJV). Now, it is important that they circumcise him on the eighth day. A lot of people are unaware, but healing has particular timing and there is a physics and frequency principle to it. The eighth element in the periodic table is oxygen and oxygen is healing.

When you turn the eight on its side, it is an infinity symbol. The infinity is known to be a protective symbol, and I actually use this movement pattern on patients. While patients are lying down, I'll move their head in a figure eight pattern and initially feel restriction in their joints and neck. But as I continue, the restriction disappears and they will begin to experience completely relaxed joint movements in their neck. So when they practice circumcision on the eighth day, it's no coincidence.

As we continue reading in Luke 1:63-64, we find that Zacharias was unable to speak because the angel told him that he would be mute. When asked for the baby's name, he writes it down. After doing so, his mouth was opened, and he was able to speak immediately (KJV). This is the power of writing.

When individuals are unable to speak, one system in the body that becomes affected is what I refer to as the lung and large intestine power line. Our body consists of various electrical systems, which I compare to power lines, linking different organ systems to the fascia, muscles, teeth, and other organs. This concept has been recognized throughout history; for instance, it can be seen in ancient practices like acupuncture and in Ayurvedic medicine, where it is associated with the chakras.

Fortunately, modern technologies have allowed us to understand these as electrical components of the body, which the ancient cultures were attempting to describe. In the case of Zacharias, it was the lung and large intestine power line that was affected.

From my observations, patients who have difficulty expressing themselves or speaking their mind often show a decrease in energy of their lung and large intestine power lines. These power lines extend from the lungs and large intestine to the upper premolars and lower molars, and they also run along the outer side of the arm to the hand.

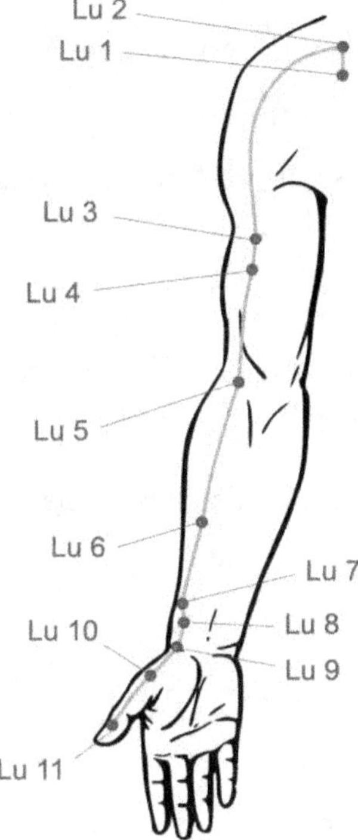

Image: "Points of lung channel de" by Dimitrius is licensed under CC BY 3.0

Although Zacharias was unable to speak, he activated the lung and large intestine power line by writing with his hand. In doing so, he expressed his voice and communicated the name of the baby, which would be John.

This is an important lesson for everyone. In today's world, many people attempt to silence others, particularly when it comes to expressing their own voices, whether online or in person. This is often seen among children in schools, where they are frequently silenced by their instructors, making it difficult to express themselves. This suppression can negatively affect the lung and large intestine power line.

When you can freely express yourself and share your thoughts, you will notice improved functioning of your lungs and large intestine. I have observed this in thousands of patients. Speaking your mind doesn't necessarily mean verbal communication; for instance, Zacharias was unable to speak, but he could express himself through writing. This highlights that both spoken and written expression can be therapeutic. In fact, individuals who engage in journaling often demonstrate higher emotional resilience.

We live in a world where darkness is trying to overshadow the light. Each individual brings their own light to the world, and we need everyone's voice. Whether it's on social media, with friends, family, in person, or through books, each perspective is of value. I encourage you to express your thoughts and feelings. By doing so, you'll find yourself feeling healthier and happier, and you will bless the lives of others.

CHAPTER 4: THE DIGITAL ROOT OF 3

In Luke 1:26-27, we read about the Angel Gabriel, who was sent by God to a virgin woman named Mary. Mary was betrothed to a man named Joseph. The text specifies that this angel was sent in the sixth month (KJV). One important principle I see in the realm of physics and numbers is a phenomenon known as the digital root of three. In this context, when you take the number six, which is essentially the number three repeated twice, it reflects the concept of the digital root of three.

Any healing number or frequency I've seen in nature will have the digital root of three. An example of one of the solfeggio frequencies is 528 Hertz. At this frequency you can calculate the digital root of three by adding the three numbers together. Two plus eight is ten, then you add five, and that equals fifteen. Then you add the one and the five from the fifteen, and that equals six, which is the digital root of three.

You see, the digital root of three will equal any combination of three, six, and nine. These are always healing numbers and healing frequencies. You will see the digital root of three show up many many times in the scriptures. Below are some of the instances I've captured, but there are likely many more.

-Matthew 1:17

-Luke 2:42

-Luke 4:25

-John 2:1, 6, 19

-John 4:6

-Luke 6:13

-Luke 11:5

-Matthew 27:9, 45

-John 21:11

-Acts 1:15

-Acts 2:15

-Acts 3:1

-Acts 10:3

-1 Timothy 5:9

-Hebrews 11:23

-Revelation 8:1

-Revelation 12:1, 6

-Revelation 14:1

-Revelation 21:12

-Revelation 22:2

I previously mentioned one of the solfeggio frequencies of 528 Hertz. This frequency is particularly beneficial for the body as it helps reduce stress (Akimoto et al., 2018). Some theorize that all music originally adhered to the solfeggio scale, including Gregorian chants; however, this connection has been lost over time. Modern music is no longer composed using this scale, which is why it is not as healing as ancient music once was.

The good news is that people are beginning to rediscover and embrace these roots.

I have seen these solfeggio frequencies significantly help entire organ systems and also help people with emotional challenges. For that reason, I have specifically calculated Solfeggio frequencies on my Healing Playbook Membership.

Now that you understand the principles of the digital root of three, you will notice this pattern everywhere, not only in the scriptures but also throughout life, especially in nature.

CHAPTER 5: FEAR, THE BLADDER POWER LINE, AND FERTILITY

In Luke 1:30-31, an angel appears to Mary and tells her that she will be the mother of Jesus (KJV). In verse 30, it's important to note that she is told to, "Fear not (KJV)." Different emotions can influence the connection between our feelings and the functioning of our body's organs. Additionally, men and women have inherent differences in their bodies for a reason.

I refer to this as masculine and feminine polarity. The body is designed like a puzzle piece, with men and women having different body parts and variations in their organ systems. Liver power lines are located around the pelvic floor area and are more dominant in men.

The bladder power line is located between the pubic bone and the belly button. This area is where a baby develops, which gives it a stronger feminine polarity. Although, this power line can be negatively influenced by the emotion of fear.

When the angel encouraged Mary to "fear not" this was promoting strength in the bladder power line.

In Luke 1:34, Mary questions how this could be possible since she knows not a man —meaning she has not been intimate with a man (KJV). Then, in verse 35, the angel responds that "the power of the Highest shall overshadow thee (KJV)." I want to emphasize the word "power."

From my observation, individuals who struggle with fertility often lack sufficient frequency or voltage in their bodies to conceive. Once people can increase the frequency and voltage within their bodies, they tend to become more fertile. This connection to the word "power" gives us additional insight into fertility.

So, what generates power in our bodies? There are several principles I have learned throughout my life and career in treating patients. First, we need to ensure that our polarities are correct. How does this occur in nature? One example is plants; they not only survive but thrive due to sunlight. One way for our bodies to retain a charge is through exposure to sunlight. I have also found that prayer, meditation, and essential oils can help correct polarity for our bodies.

To actually charge the body, several methods can be effective. Acts of kindness, reading scripture, and grounding—such as placing your bare feet on grass, dirt, or sand—are beneficial. Additionally, exercise is crucial; when we move our muscles, they generate frequency, which travels through a layer of tissue called fascia and connects with different parts of the body. Sound can also generate frequencies that aid in recharging the body.

Therefore, if you are struggling with fertility, using these various methods can not only help your body hold a charge but also provide it with enough power to become fertile.

CHAPTER 6: MOVEMENT IN PREGNANCY

In Luke 1:39-41, it says that Mary arose and she "went into the hill country with haste (KJV)."

There is a special meaning in the phrase "with haste." It doesn't just state that she traveled to the hill country; it emphasizes that she did so with energy.

There's a special meaning to the role of mothers in the health and energy of their babies, simply through movement. Some of the healthiest people I've known, of various ages, are those who move frequently and with speed. When we think about the Savior, it's remarkable to consider all He accomplished in His life. One can't help but reflect on the example of His mother, who, while pregnant, passed on energy to Him through her own movement.

I find that one of the best things women can do during pregnancy is to exercise. It doesn't have to be anything intense; simple activities like walking can suffice. Unfortunately, in today's world, many people lead sedentary lifestyles, which can also negatively impact the baby. When pregnant women are able to get out and move more, their babies tend to be healthier.

There's also a spiritual principle at play here. When Mary visited Elisabeth, the baby leaped in her womb at the sound of Mary's voice. This illustrates two important points: our words and presence are healing. We all possess something called a biofield, an energy field that extends about five or six feet from our bodies. If you've ever entered a room with someone without speaking or touching them, you might have felt their energy—whether good or bad—emanating from their biofield. Everyone has one. Mary's good energy was felt not only through her voice but also through her presence.

When we radiate good and positive energy, we help those around us feel better. When people feel good, they are more aware of the Holy Spirit in their lives. Some of the most inspiring individuals I've encountered are high-energy people. In our current world, we need leaders, and effective leaders are often those with energy. To increase energy in your life, movement is key. It is not just beneficial for you; the world around you needs it too.

CHAPTER 7: CHALLENGING CHILDREN'S IMMUNE SYSTEMS AND FIBONACCI

In Luke 2:4-7, we read about the birth of Jesus Christ. Verse 7 specifically mentions that Mary wrapped the Savior in swaddling clothes and laid Him in a manger (KJV). This detail carries an important principle relevant to our lives today: the manger, a place where animals eat, symbolizes His ultimate sacrifice for us. When we consider the Savior's healing capabilities, we see how He embodies the challenge to our immune systems. The manger was likely dirty, yet Mary did not shy away from it; she actually embraced the opportunity to challenge her son's immune system.

In our day, many children miss out on this exposure. Since 2020, many have become germaphobic, including parents who are overly protective of their children. However, there's something beneficial about allowing kids to challenge their immune systems. When we overly protect our children, their immune systems may not learn to fight off germs effectively. I've noticed that individuals who have had significant exposure to germs often turn out to be some of the healthiest people I know. It's essential for children to spend time outdoors, play with other kids, and learn how to navigate their environments. The earlier they do this, the stronger their immune systems will be as they grow.

We later learn that the Savior was circumcised on the eighth day, and this timing holds significance. Previously, we read that the number eight symbolizes oxygen, which is associated with healing. Additionally, eight is a Fibonacci number, a key pattern in the universe.

The Fibonacci sequence builds upon itself, where each number is the sum of the two preceding ones. Here's how the Fibonacci sequence works:

- Start with 0 and 1.
- $0 + 1 = 1$.
- Then, take the two previous numbers (1 and 0) and add them together: $1 + 0 = 1$.
- Next, add the last two numbers (1 and 1): $1 + 1 = 2$.
- Now, add the most recent two numbers (1 and 2): $1 + 2 = 3$.
- Continue with the next set (2 and 3): $2 + 3 = 5$.
- Finally, add these two (3 and 5): $3 + 5 = 8$.

This sequence manifests a repeated pattern in nature, such as in seashells, hurricanes, and waves. Fibonacci numbers are not only a mathematical concept; they are also believed to have healing properties. They relate to scalar waves, which are a different type of waveform compared to electromagnetic waves.

While electromagnetic waves are linear and move up and down, scalar waves are known as longitudinal waves, which curve instead. Interestingly, the structure of the DNA helix follows a Fibonacci pattern. By applying the principles of Fibonacci and incorporating the digital root of 3, we can discover various effective healing methods.

CHAPTER 8: THE WISE MEN, STARS, GOLD, FRANKINCENSE, MYRRH, EGYPT, AND ISRAEL

In Matthew 2:1-2, we read about wise men coming from the East who followed a star to worship the King of the Jews (KJV). This illustrates an important principle: these wise men must have been very successful individuals. We will explore why that is significant later.

Historically, many ancient people used the stars for navigation, which required them to look up at the sky frequently. Looking up is a powerful principle that we seem to have lost in our modern world. Today, many spend their time looking down at their phones. This not only affects their view of the world but also harms their posture. Our cervical spine and neck are designed to have a natural curve, and I am noticing more and more young people developing a forward head posture due to this trend.

Good posture is crucial for health and confidence. Individuals with better posture not only experience physical benefits but also project greater self-assurance. Research indicates that people are naturally drawn to those with good posture.

In addition to posture, spending time outdoors is incredibly beneficial to our health. Historically, people had to go outside for various aspects of daily life. In contrast, many of us today find ourselves confined indoors due to work, school, and commuting. However, going outside—even at night—allows exposure to infrared light. This type of light, which can come from the moon and stars, has healing properties.

When we think about water, we typically recognize three states: solid, liquid, and gas. However, Gerald Pollack presents compelling evidence for a fourth phase of water. Water has the chemical formula H_2O, which consists of two hydrogen atoms and one oxygen atom. Dr. Pollack has shown that when water is exposed to infrared light, it transforms into a structured or "charged" form known as H_3O_2, which contains three hydrogen atoms and two oxygen atoms. This new structure can have healing effects, suggesting that we should spend more time outdoors. While daytime exposure is ideal, nighttime exposure is also beneficial (Pollack).

In Matthew 2:11, we learn that the wise men brought gifts of gold, frankincense, and myrrh when they visited the Christ child (KJV). Each of these gifts holds special significance. Gold, for instance, has always retained its value over time, not only for its monetary worth but also for its healing properties. The color and composition of gold emit strong vibrations that can positively influence health.

Frankincense has a distinctive frequency because of its monoterpenes, which resonate with the spleen, stomach, and pancreas power line.

On the other hand, myrrh contains sesquiterpenes that resonate with four specific power lines: the lungs, large intestine, kidneys, and bladder.

We will soon explore why these power lines are significant to the Savior and His family.

In Matthew 2:13-15, we see that after the wise men departed, an angel of the Lord appeared to Joseph in a dream. The angel instructed him to take Jesus, the Savior, and His mother to flee to Egypt (KJV). There is a specific reason why the angel mentioned Egypt. Throughout history, certain places on Earth have been recognized as high-energy locations, and Bethlehem and Egypt are two examples.

Ancient Egypt was notable for many remarkable discoveries, and God's dealings often occurred there. For instance, Abraham had roots in Egypt, Joseph was sold into Egypt, Joseph's family later moved there, and Moses led the Israelites out of Egypt. Many significant historical events unfolded in this region.

The pyramids of Egypt are particularly impressive and have withstood the test of time. In fact, our modern technology cannot reproduce the engineering feats accomplished in constructing the pyramids. While many consider these structures to be tombs, locals believe that the pyramids were actually power generators.

The pyramids are constructed as geometric shapes known as Platonic solids. They are associated with scalar energy, which operates on a different waveform than sunlight. Scalar energy tends to create vortex patterns that can form shapes like pyramids. The pyramids were built using specific materials and designed with particular shapes to harness these energies effectively.

When you examine some of the murals in Egypt, it appears that figures are holding items that resemble light bulbs.

Several colleagues of mine who have visited Egypt have noted an interesting observation: when you look up at certain ancient structures, you can see that there is no soot on the walls. Typically, when fires burn, they leave behind black or brown residue.

However, in some of these Egyptian sites, there is an absence of this soot. This raises a question: if the ancient Egyptians did not burn fires and the structures lacked windows, how did they illuminate the interiors of places like the pyramids?

It is now theorized that the ancient Egyptians may have had access to a form of electricity. This idea is supported by the depictions in the murals where figures appear to be holding what look like light bulbs.

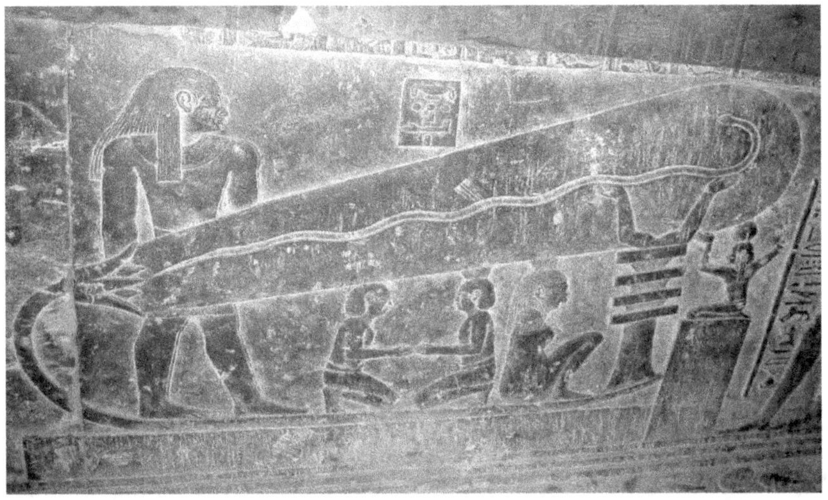

Image: "Dendera03.jpg" By Rowan is licensed under CC BY 4.0

Some of these chambers, along with certain Egyptian pyramids, exhibit perfect harmonics. It is believed that they may have been used for healing purposes through sound in these acoustically ideal rooms. Therefore, I think the Savior may have benefited from the environment. While he is undoubtedly the greatest source of this power, I truly believe in the significance of these harmonics.

Our circumstances influence us, which is why I believe the angel specifically instructed them to go to Egypt.

Another interesting aspect is the inspiration that the wise men had in presenting gifts to the Savior and his family.

The first gift was gold. I consider gold to be a high-frequency material, which is why it has maintained its value over time. The second gift was frankincense. I previously mentioned that the monoterpenes in frankincense resonate with the spleen, stomach, and pancreas power lines.

These power lines not only affect those specific organs but also influence other connected organs. In addition to the spleen, stomach, and pancreas, this power line also connects to the thyroid, adrenals, and reproductive organs.

When you have a power line that maintains good frequency and vibration, it positively influences other organs as well.

Additionally, emotions can affect these organs, and one that impacts this power line is worry. For instance, when Joseph dreamt of an angel telling him to flee to Egypt, it's likely that worry was one of the emotions he felt. Interestingly, they had frankincense with them.

Frankincense can help alleviate feelings of worry. Also, having to escape from a situation triggers the body's fight or flight response. During stressful moments, it is crucial to support the adrenal glands. Therefore, having frankincense not only helped them manage their emotions but also supported their adrenal and thyroid glands, providing the energy needed for their journey.

They were also given myrrh, which contains sesquiterpenes that resonate with the lung, large intestine, kidney, and bladder power line.

The lungs and large intestine also contribute energy to the nasal septum.

Furthermore, the kidneys and bladder power the occipital lobe of the brain and the corpus callosum, which connects the two hemispheres of the brain, as well as the frontal sinuses.

Grief affects the lungs and large intestine, while fear impacts the kidneys and bladder. When the wise men presented myrrh to the Savior and his family, it likely provided them with emotional support. Leaving home can evoke a profound sense of grief, and it's understandable that they may have felt fear as well.

Given that Egypt is a dry, hot place, characterized by frequent dust storms, maintaining healthy mucous membranes would have been crucial for them. The myrrh would have supported not just their frontal sinuses, but also the salivary glands in a dry desert.

This is amazing, and it's no coincidence that the wise men provided these gifts.

Ultimately, these gifts symbolize the Savior himself and his healing power.

All healing is possible because of Him and through Him. He paid the price for everyone's sins and pains. When He suffered in the Garden of Gethsemane, He felt the pain that everyone in this world has ever experienced. It is because of Him that we are healed. From the foundation of His life, having strong roots and beginnings was essential for Him to bear the pains and sins of the world.

In Matthew 2:19, we learn that Herod has died, and an angel appears to Joseph in a dream. In verse 20, the angel instructs him to take Jesus and His mother and return to Israel (KJV).

I previously mentioned that Egypt is a high-frequency place, but Israel is also significant in this regard. It's no surprise that Christians, Jewish, and Muslims gather in Israel. Not only does the location hold spiritual significance, but there is also a strong frequency and vibration there that promotes healing.

CHAPTER 9: FEMININE POLARITY, THE HEART, AND INCREASING IN STATURE

In Luke 2:19,51, it says that Mary both pondered and kept these things in her heart (KJV). We previously discussed how different power lines in the body can have either masculine or feminine polarity.

The heart and small intestine power lines specifically embody feminine energy, which makes sense considering that breast tissue protrudes outward in women, where this power line occurs right in the middle of the chest. When women draw upon their feminine energy, it positively influences both their bodies and minds, particularly in practices like pondering and meditation. These activities help correct polarity in the body, allowing it to better hold a charge. Additionally, this connection creates feelings of joy, which is associated with the heart power line.

Women have a wonderful opportunity to share their joy with those around them, especially mothers who can teach their children valuable lessons. In Luke 2:52, it states that Jesus grew "in wisdom and stature, and in favour with God and man (KJV)".

This principle is particularly important for us today. Children are exposed to so much information now, perhaps more than ever, but I notice that they are not growing in stature as much as past generations, especially when compared to the Savior. In the times when Jesus lived, movement was essential to daily life.

Today, many people are not as physically active. This sedentary lifestyle negatively impacts both mental and physical health, which in turn affects growth.

Reflecting on my own childhood, I remember spending a lot of time outdoors, running around, and participating in physical education (PE) classes and recess. Unfortunately, schools have reduced the time allocated for PE and recess, leading to a concerning trend. Many kids now come home and opt to watch TV, play video games, or use computers instead of playing outside with friends.

While these activities aren't inherently bad, it's crucial to remember that everything should be done in moderation. Lack of physical activity can hinder growth—mentally, physically, spiritually, and emotionally. The Savior accomplished so much in his life—he traveled extensively, healed the sick, and taught others—all of which required movement.

If we encourage kids to be active from a young age, we can help them develop healthier habits and set them up for success in life.

CHAPTER 10: PERFECTIONISM AND DOVES

In John 1:27, we read about John the Baptist. While he was preaching, he made it clear to the people that the person coming after him, referring to the Savior, was preferred before him and that he was not worthy to unloose the latch of his shoes (KJV).

When John expresses this, it highlights a tendency many people, including myself, have: perfectionism in thinking. Perfectionism can be very dangerous for our minds and bodies.

After this moment, the Savior did come to John the Baptist, and even though John believed he wasn't worthy to unlatch his shoe, the Savior needed him to baptize Him as an example for all of us. Therefore, John was indeed worthy to perform that act.

I have also struggled with perfectionism in my thinking, and I've noticed that when I fall into this mindset, I am not as happy mentally.

This issue is amplified by social media. Today, social media can be a double-edged sword; it can be used for good but can also have harmful effects. I strive to focus on using it positively, but many people fall into the trap of comparing themselves to others because of social media. This comparison can lead to two extremes: feeling superior, which breeds pride, or feeling inferior, which leads to sadness.

The reality is that when we look at social media, we often see only the best, most perfect moments of people's lives, unaware that many are struggling behind the scenes. It can take hundreds of pictures to get just one that looks perfect. We don't see the effort that goes into creating that one ideal image or video.

Everything in life requires effort, but when we obsess over perfection for ourselves or others, we overlook the higher law that Christ embodies. He makes up for all our shortcomings. He serves as the mediator for us spiritually, physically, mentally, and emotionally.

We do not have to be perfect in this life because perfection is unattainable here; it comes after this life, and only through the Savior, Jesus Christ, is it possible. His message to John and to all of us is that even if we feel we are not perfect, we are enough. He makes all the difference, and if we turn to Him, He can help us become better than we ever imagined.

Additionally, in John 1:32, we read that after John the Baptist baptized Jesus, he saw the Spirit descend from heaven like a dove (KJV).

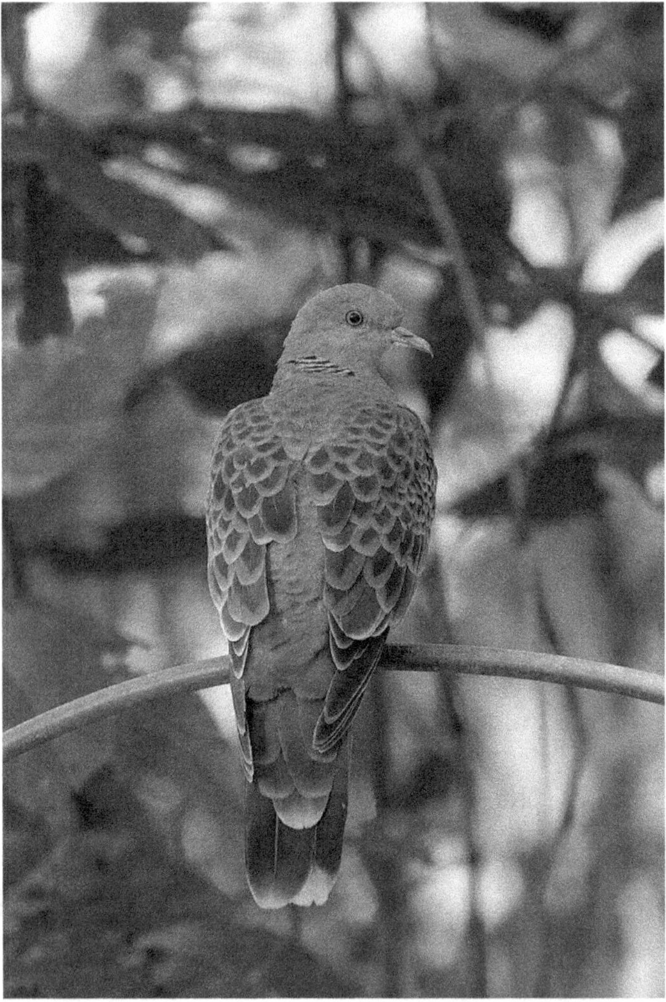

Image: "Oriental turtle dove by Tisha Mukherjee 02.jpg" By Tisha Mukherjee is licensed under CC BY 4.0

It is no coincidence that the word "dove" was used to describe this event. Doves produce an audible frequency range of 210 to 1100 Hertz (Cate, 2004). This resonates with every organ and power line of the body, promoting healing when you hear a dove coo.

Anytime we invite the Spirit into our lives, it brings healing and increases our frequency and vibration. Therefore, by inviting the Spirit through gospel music, reading scriptures, praying, going to church, serving others, and keeping the commandments, we enhance our overall well-being.

CHAPTER 11: STONES

In John 1:42, Simon, the son of Jonah, was brought to the Savior, who called him Cephas, meaning "a stone (KJV)." While many people often view stones as mere objects, each stone carries its own unique vibration and frequency, much like crystals. Referring to Simon as a "stone" can be interpreted as a compliment, acknowledging his potential as a healer. Although he may not yet recognize this potential, with the Lord's help, he can achieve great things.

I have personally used various stones and crystals and have observed their benefits when cut in certain patterns and frequency from either light or sound passing through them onto patients, and my findings have been remarkable.

These crystals can generate what is known as scalar frequencies. There is also electromagnetic frequency, or transverse waves, which move linearly up and down. In contrast, scalar waves exhibit a vortex-like motion; they expand outward and converge at a single point, similar to a DNA helix.

When a specific wavelength of light passes through a crystal cut to particular dimensions and shapes, it transforms the light into scalar waves. Applying these waves to the body can help correct a phenomenon known as polarity. The human body can be likened to stacks of rechargeable batteries. When the body's energy drops to zero, the positive and negative charges can become inverted. By introducing scalar frequencies to the body, polarity can be restored, enabling the body to hold a charge effectively.

I have also applied brainwave frequencies through scalar waves and have observed positive effects in almost every case. The brain is responsible for spatial awareness, which can be tested using what I call the cerebellum finger-to-nose test. In this test, a patient extends their finger in a specific direction with their eyes open and then returns it to their nose. If they struggle to find their finger after closing their eyes three times, it may indicate a lack of spatial awareness.

After using scalar frequencies derived from crystals, I retest the patient and often find that the brain can now accurately locate the body in space. Many people notice improvements in their posture, while athletes report enhanced performance in activities like basketball and weightlifting.

Unfortunately, many crystals and stones have lost their beneficial frequencies due to radiation or heat treatment. Such treatments can diminish a crystal's vibrational quality, rendering it ineffective for healing.

We will explore different stones and crystals mentioned in the New Testament later, but it's essential to remember that these natural elements possess healing qualities. One way to elevate your frequency is by touching various rocks and stones in nature, which can serve as a grounding technique, even without being near grass, sand, or dirt. That is also why I created my own scalar frequency device that I call the Infinity light that uses these principles and uses crystals without radiation that are cut in geometrical patterns to increase scalar frequencies. I have seen this benefit numerous patients and device owners. One practitioner claims they see symptoms improve in as fast as 5 seconds. That is the power of scalar frequencies.

CHAPTER 12: THE TORUS FIELD OF TREES AND FIGS

Nathaniel came to the Savior and was surprised when the Savior told him that He had seen him. In John 1:47-48, it mentions that Jesus saw Nathaniel under a fig tree (KJV). The Savior is the ultimate master of waveforms, and when Nathaniel was under the fig tree, he was in the presence of this powerful energy.

Whether you are touching a tree or simply nearby, you are actually receiving energy from it. There is a phenomenon called a toroidal field, and the human body, as I previously mentioned, also forms a toroidal shape. This energy field is small in the center and expands outward, curving back in to become small again.

Trees exhibit this toroidal pattern; you can see it in their structure—the main trunk is small, and then it branches out towards the leaves. This energy flows outward and continues to branch out as it reaches the roots. Finally, it returns to the trunk. Similarly, the human body has this pattern. The trunk of our bodies—our core, which includes our stomach and back—resembles the trunk of a tree.

Energy radiates outward and circulates between our head, arms, and back, returning from our legs to our trunk. When you touch a tree, you receive electrons, but when you are beneath a tree's branches, you also absorb frequencies.

The Savior, being the creator of this world, is the master of wavelengths and is aware of people near high-frequency objects. In our time, we can relate to this by resting against trees or being near them. Trees not only promote healing and health in humans but also offer protection. I have seen trees surrounding a house transmute harmful electromagnetic energy, such as EMFs.

Figs themselves are also very healthy. Fig trees have a variety of chemical compositions that resonate with different organ systems which include phenolics, sesquiterpenes, monoterpenes, and alcohols (Mawa et al., 2013). The phenolics align with the heart and small intestine power lines, sesquiterpenes that connect with the kidney, bladder, lung, and large intestine power lines, and monoterpenes resonate with the spleen, stomach, and pancreas power lines. Additionally, they contain alcohols that correlate with both the parasympathetic and sympathetic power lines, making figs what I consider to be a superfood.

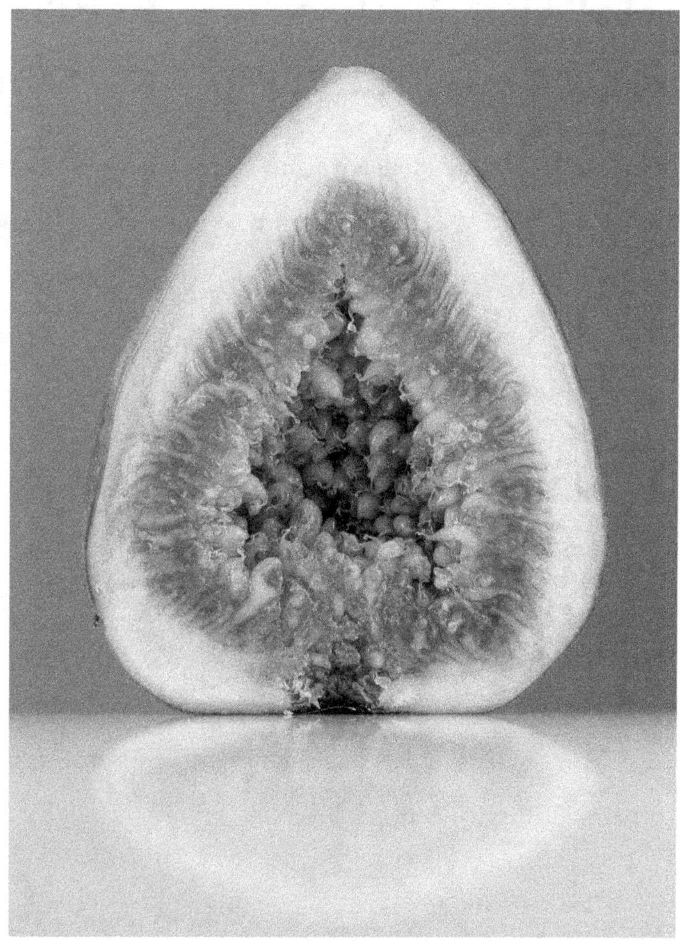

Image: "Fig (Ficus carica) fruit halved.jpg" By Ivar Leidus is licensed under CC BY 4.0

CHAPTER 13: JOHN THE BAPTIST, CAMEL'S HAIR, LOCUSTS, AND HONEY

In Matthew 3:1-4, we read about John the Baptist preaching in the wilderness of Judea. It is noted that he wore camel's hair and that his diet consisted of locusts and honey (KJV). There are several health principles we can derive from this.

First, the wilderness surrounding Judea is predominantly desert, which suggests that adapting to our local environments involves using locally sourced products. This is one reason why John the Baptist wore camel's hair. Camels are well-adapted to thrive in dry heat, so wearing materials that are local to our environment can enhance our frequency and vibration while also helping us acclimate. More natural materials, such as cotton, wool, and leather, tend to be healthier for our bodies.

Unfortunately, in today's world, many synthetic materials can lower our frequency and vibration. The only situation in which I believe synthetic materials are acceptable is during survival scenarios, such as long backpacking or camping trips. In those cases, polyester dries quickly and can aid in survival. However, for everyday clothing, it's better to opt for natural materials.

Dr. Max Collins, a prestigious mentor of mine, is an expert in health and endurance. He has extensive experience hiking diverse terrains. In my conversations with him, he has emphasized that synthetic materials can be beneficial in survival situations. Natural fabrics, on the other hand, are preferable for daily wear.

We can also learn from John the Baptist's diet of locusts and honey. In the wilderness, food and water options are limited, so consuming local foods can benefit one's health. There is some debate regarding the term "locust"; some suggest he may have eaten from the locust tree. This tree is found in hotter, drier climates and is considered toxic, yet it resembles a pea.

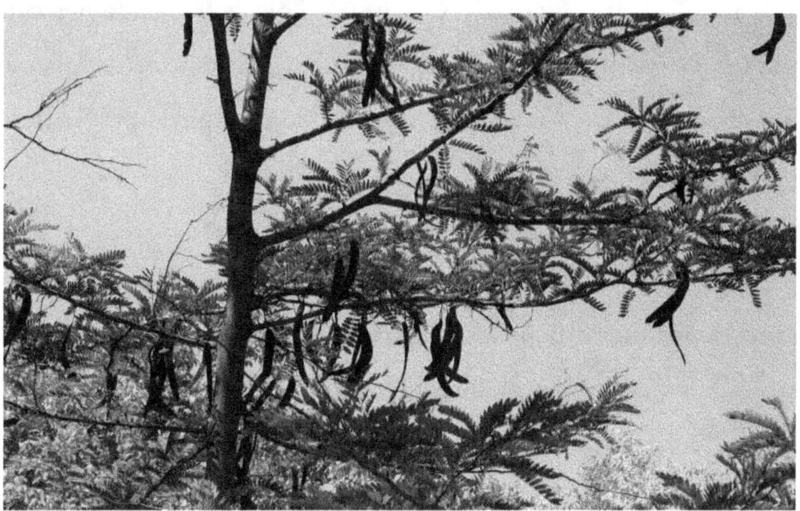

Image: "Honey locust (Gleditsia tiacanthos) branches" By Humoyun Mehridinov is licensed under CC BY 4.0

If he did eat from the locust tree, the addition of honey could aid in fermenting and making these foods more digestible.

Alternatively, if he consumed actual locusts, there is a frequency principle we can derive from this. The wings of locusts produce a beat frequency ranging from 10 to 26 Hertz (Kutsch, 1973). Interestingly, this frequency is believed to transfer through food, resonating with alpha and beta brainwave patterns known to promote mental clarity and learning.

Honey also carries its own frequencies. Bees create a buzzing sound with a frequency range of 100 to 300 Hertz, which can even jump to 500 to 600 Hertz (Ferrari et al., 2008). This frequency range can help alleviate pain and inflammation and is relevant to the spleen, stomach, and pancreas. The adrenals are on the spleen power line, which assist in body temperature regulation and would have been beneficial for John the Baptist living in a hot wilderness.

Furthermore, the structure of beehives, which resemble platonic solids, allows scalar energy from the sun to accumulate, enhancing their frequency. The hexagonal shape of the hive, featuring six sides, connects to healing numbers, such as the digital root of 3, which appears frequently in nature.

Thus, just as John the Baptist did, if we consume foods and wear materials that are unique to our local environment, it can enhance our frequency and vibration, ultimately supporting our health.

CHAPTER 14: STONES, THE LIVER, AND TESTOSTERONE

In Matthew 3:9, it says that God is able to raise up children unto Abraham from these stones. The term "stones" can be understood in two different ways (KJV).

First, stones represent grounding. When we consider the body's power lines, the liver power line is a key grounding element. This power line begins at the bottom of the big toe and ascends along the inside of the leg and thigh, reaching up to the pelvic floor, next to where the male genitals are located. This leads us to the second interpretation of "raising up children": the stones could also refer to the testis.

In the next verse, Matthew 3:10, it states that the axe is laid to the root of the tree. I want to emphasize the "root of the tree" here because it combines principles from various ancient practices, including Oriental and Ayurvedic medicine. We know that the liver's power line runs from the bottom of the toe to the inside of the thigh, which is exactly where the liver meridian in traditional acupuncture is located.

In Ayurvedic medicine, there is a concept known as the root chakra, represented by the color red. I've observed that patients with liver problems often wear red, even though they are not conscious of this, I believe it is to help their body. This principle is observed in various ancient medical techniques and is also reflected in scripture. It's known in Oriental medicine that wood is associated with the liver meridian. I refer to this as the "power line" because modern principles allow us to connect these ancient ideas to contemporary understanding.

The mention of trees in this context is significant because trees are made of wood. The rest of Matthew 3:10 states that trees that do not produce good fruit are cut down and cast into the fire (KJV). Many people may associate this solely with having children; indeed, one of our life goals is to produce offspring who are as successful, if not more so, than we are.

One factor that aids in the production of children is testosterone. There are two power lines involved in testosterone production, and one of them originates from the liver power line, which is connected to the root chakra located between the legs where the male genitals descend. However, this is not limited to having children. Increased testosterone levels also provide us with drive and energy.

With more drive and energy, we can achieve more in life, in business, and in serving others. Testosterone boosts our energy levels, and when we have sufficient energy flowing through the liver power line, we will produce more testosterone. This not only enhances fertility but also empowers us to make a positive impact in the world.

CHAPTER 15: 40 DAYS IN THE WILDERNESS

In Mark 1:12-13, it states that the Savior was driven by the Spirit into the wilderness, where He was tempted by the adversary. He was among wild beasts but was also ministered to by angels (KJV). He spent 40 days there, a duration that carries special significance, which we will discuss later.

Being in the wilderness for such an extended time must have been a humbling experience. Although the Savior was accustomed to living in humble circumstances, such as being born in a stable and lying in a manger, this period in the wilderness had its challenges.

Dr. Max Collins frequently speaks of his experiences on long hikes that last for weeks at a time. He has mentioned that these lengthy treks are incredibly humbling. Humility is beneficial for one's health; it encourages self-improvement and simplifies life. We will explore the concept of simplicity in more detail in a future chapter.

The Savior's 40-day trek in the wilderness served as a mentally, spiritually, and emotionally healing experience, as well as a physically revitalizing one. Dr. Collins has noted that long expeditions can tone the body and provide physical cleansing through movement.

There is also deep significance in the number 40, which occurs frequently in scripture. Interestingly, 40 Hz is a frequency that can help neural activity (Suk et al., 2023), and it is one of the frequencies I utilize in my membership program with great success. This correlation between the number 40 and memory is meaningful, as I mentioned earlier, all healing comes through the Savior, Jesus Christ. There are numbers that point to Him, and 40 is one of them. When you listen to 40 Hz, which supports memory, it can also serve as a reminder of the Savior as the ultimate healer.

CHAPTER 16: THE LEPER, TOUCH, WORDS, AND THE LARGE INTESTINE

In Mark 1:40, it says that a leper came to the Savior and knelt before Him (KJV). Kneeling is an interesting practice that we often see in prayer, and it also has the effect of raising our frequency. When you place your feet on natural materials like grass, dirt, or sand, you connect with the Earth and draw power from it.

When you kneel, both of your feet and your knees are in contact with the ground, which enhances your connection to the Earth and increases your power. Thus, the act of kneeling not only demonstrates humility before the Savior but also elevates your personal energy.

In Mark 1:40-42, the leper asked to be cleansed and healed by the Savior. In response, the Savior reached out His hand and told him to be healed, and he was indeed healed (KJV).

Leprosy is a serious skin condition that can severely damage the skin and even cause limbs to fall off. Many skin conditions arise from low power in the large intestine's power line. When the large intestine becomes inflamed and overly acidic, it struggles to eliminate toxins and inflammation from the body. As a result, the body is forced to expel these toxins through the skin, which could explain my suspicion that leprosy is linked to low power in the large intestine.

When the Savior extended His hand and spoke, we learn two important principles related to frequency. First, the power line of the large intestine connects to the upper part of the body, particularly around the thumb area. So when the Savior touched the leper, He was transmitting healing power from his body.

Secondly, speaking is also a form of frequency. The vocal aspect of healing ties into the lung-large intestine in Ayurvedic medicine, which is related to the throat chakra. I like to modernize this concept by referring to it as the lung-large intestine power line.

When people emotionally struggle to express themselves, it decreases the power in the lung and large intestine. This is significant because when the Savior used both His hands to touch the leper and His voice to speak healing, He effectively utilized two different principles of frequency. He exemplifies the ultimate healer, which is why the leper was cured.

Physical touch has healing capabilities, a fact that has been overlooked in recent years. Many people have become fearful of physical contact due to concerns of germs and illness. However, physical touch is vital; for instance, holding hands with someone completes a circuit that enhances the energy in both individuals.

Additionally, when someone with a stronger energy field touches someone with a weaker one, the person with greater power can transfer some of that power to the other. This is particularly helpful for someone who is sick or injured, as they can receive healing energy from the person with more power. Ultimately, the Savior, having the most power of anyone to ever exist, is the reason why so many people were healed, including this leper.

CHAPTER 17: MINIMALIST LIFESTYLE

In Luke 3:11-13, the Savior teaches that those who have two coats should share with those who have none and to not demand more than what is appointed to them (KJV). This can be seen as a lesson in generosity, but it also promotes a minimalist lifestyle. Additionally, 1 Corinthians 14:40 instructs us to let all things be done decently and in order, while 1 Corinthians 14:33 reminds us that "God is not the author of confusion, but of peace (KJV)."

In our daily lives, we often find ourselves surrounded by an abundance of material possessions, yet these things do not bring true happiness. I have discovered that embracing minimalist principles leads to greater contentment. So, what exactly is a minimalist lifestyle? It is the practice of keeping only what you truly need.

When it comes to accumulating wealth, I believe it is acceptable to earn money, provided it is done ethically and used for good. However, gathering material possessions that go unused does not lead to fulfillment. Many people continuously seek the latest and greatest items, believing that these objects will bring happiness. In reality, true happiness comes from the Gospel of Jesus Christ, not from material things.

For me, a minimalist lifestyle means focusing on the essential aspects of life that contribute to overall happiness and well-being. These core needs include a relationship with God, connections with family and friends, and having a home, clothing, food, and health. The more we simplify our lives, the happier we can become.

I witnessed this principle firsthand while growing up. I spent countless hours watching television, always searching for the next best show or movie, but often ended up feeling disappointed. A couple of years ago, we decided to get rid of our TV, which forced us to embrace a more minimalist lifestyle. This was one of the best decisions we ever made. Not only did we accomplish more, but I also noticed that our family members were happier. Without a TV, we became more creative and active.

One effective way to simplify and enhance our lives is by organizing our living spaces. When we accumulate too much clutter and lack organization, it creates chaos that can make it difficult to feel the spirit in our homes. The Lord encourages simplicity and order.

This simplicity applies not only to the possessions we hold but also to the stress that arises from being overly committed. Many people experience significant stress from juggling too many activities, impacting their health. By simplifying our commitments, we can genuinely enjoy what we do, bringing joy to our minds, bodies, and spirits.

By embracing simplicity in both our schedules and our homes, we can experience a better flow in life and greater happiness, allowing us to invite the spirit more fully into our lives. This approach helps us be more present and appreciate the wonderful gifts the Lord has given us. Often, we focus too much on material possessions, but true happiness comes from faith, family, good health, and having a place to call home.

In our modern culture, these may seem like small or simple things, but when we take the time to truly enjoy the presence of our loved ones and savor the simple moments, life becomes significantly more fulfilling. If you are seeking a simpler lifestyle that promotes happiness, consider exploring a minimalist lifestyle.

CHAPTER 18: PALSY, GUILT, FORGIVENESS, AND TAKING ACTION

In Luke 5:24-25, Jesus Christ approaches a man with palsy and tells him "that the Son of Man hath power upon earth to forgive sins (KJV)."

This passage teaches us an important principle about sin. When we sin—knowingly go against what God desires for us—we distance ourselves from Him. God is the ultimate healer and embodies the highest frequency and vibration, such qualities we aspire to emulate. When we fail to align with God's will, we lower our own frequency and vibration, which can lead to sickness.

It's essential to note, however, that this does not imply that everyone who experiences sickness or injury has distanced themselves from God. We live in a fallen world governed by natural laws, and violating these laws can result in illness. Yet, the closer we draw to God, especially through our Savior, Jesus Christ, the happier and healthier we can become.

Guilt is a significant burden for many people. In my experience working with patients facing emotional difficulties, I have observed that those unable to forgive others often struggle with overwhelming emotions. While I am not the judge of anyone's experiences—only God can judge—those who have a willingness to forgive, even if challenging at first, can gradually find relief. Practicing forgiveness in our thoughts, words, and actions can raise our own frequency and vibration.

Often, the hardest person to forgive is ourselves. In a world that promotes perfectionism, especially through social media where people showcase their best moments, it's easy to forget that everyone has faced challenges. We all make mistakes, so it's important not to be too hard on ourselves. God is always proud of you and wants you to thrive and be happy.

Focus on doing your best to improve each day; God cares about your effort and willingness. This is a crucial aspect of the Savior's healing moments—spiritual healing paired with actionable guidance. For example, the Savior directed the man with palsy to "arise, take up thy couch, and go into thine house." This illustrates a vital principle about action.

In our healthcare culture, there is often an unrealistic expectation that healing should happen instantaneously, like taking a magic pill. While the Savior can heal in an instant, we must acknowledge that we currently live in a fallen world. I believe that when He returns, all will be made well instantly, but in our present reality, healing usually requires time and action.

Faith without works is dead. It's not enough to believe you can be healed; you also need to take action. For someone with palsy, it would be easy to think they should be overly cautious after healing. However, the Savior commanded him to stand, take up his bed, and move, emphasizing the importance of action. Movement is crucial to our health and wellbeing.

When examining the effects of an inactive lifestyle, I find that being confined to a bed, either as a patient or a caregiver, can be draining. Encouraging movement, even in small amounts when one is sick or injured, is vital. Physical activity not only energizes the body but also positively affects mental and emotional health.

Interestingly, muscles and fascia are piezoelectric, meaning that movement generates frequencies within our bodies that provide energy. Furthermore, movement helps support our lymphatic systems, which function as the body's sewage system, removing toxins and inflammation from organs and tissues.

I appreciate how the Savior encouraged action. In my practice, I always provide patients with something to do. I often say you can either fish for someone or teach them how to fish. The Savior's approach teaches others how to fish, fostering independence and resilience.

CHAPTER 19: CLOTHING AND HARMFUL FREQUENCIES

In Luke 5:36, it says that the Savior mentioned that no one puts a piece of new garment onto an old one. If they do, the piece taken from the new garment will not agree with the old (KJV).

This concept highlights an interesting principle related to clothing. Different materials can absorb harmful energy, which we've discussed before in relation to emotions. Traumatic events can lead to emotional experiences that get stored in our bodies, draining our power. Similarly, these emotions can be transferred to our clothing.

When you go to work or encounter a stressful situation, you may not be consciously aware of it, but many people instinctively change their clothes upon returning home. This act serves as a way to prevent the frequency of any stressful experiences from lingering on their bodies.

I have observed this principle time and time again. Fortunately, just because you experience a stressful event doesn't mean the negative energy will remain in your clothes forever. One effective way to eliminate this build-up of harmful frequencies is by washing them.

This concept is practical for everyday life, though it can be taken to extremes if misapplied. It's impractical to wash your clothes every time you experience stress. Instead, using natural materials like cotton, linen, and wool can be beneficial, as they tend to absorb less harmful frequencies compared to synthetic fabrics.

Color schemes also play a role; darker colors are known to absorb more harmful frequencies. However, certain colors can help with specific emotions, which we will discuss in the future.

It's fascinating that the Savior pointed out in scripture that when you combine new clothing with old, there is potential for harmful frequencies to transfer. Washing your clothes can help eliminate this. This principle allows us to better understand the phenomenon we observe in everyday life concerning frequency and scripture.

CHAPTER 20: FERMENTATION AND DIGESTION

Luke 5:39 says, "No man also having drunk old wine straightway desireth new: for he saith, The old is better (KJV)."

As I mentioned previously, I don't believe our bodies were meant to drink alcohol. However, during the time of Christ, there weren't many sources of clean water available. We are fortunate to live in an era where clean water is accessible to most people.

In those days, people drank wine because it was typically fermented grape juice and one of the few clean sources of liquid. When it is said that "the old is better," I believe this refers to fermentation as a general principle.

When considering modern diets, humans are not 100% herbivores or 100% carnivores; we are omnivores. This means we need our food to be broken down effectively. I learned this principle also from Dr. Max Collins, and it has always resonated with me, particularly when I was unwell.

Initially, I didn't understand much about diet and its role in our health, but I discovered that increasing my intake of probiotics was vital for my well-being. We obtain probiotics from fermented foods, such as sauerkraut and kimchi. However, it's not just limited to these; pickled foods work well too—like pickles, pickled onions, and pickled jalapeños. These foods are created by soaking ingredients in vinegar, salt, or acidic substances like lemon or lime juice to preserve them.

Unfortunately, many foods today are preserved with artificial preservatives, which can be toxic because they are foreign to our bodies. In contrast, natural fermentation and pickling processes are healthy. I remember a time when my family saw an apple cider vinegar that was past its expiration date. Dr. Collins pointed out that even though it was expired, it was better because it had fermented longer.

The longer the fermentation, the more probiotics it contains. This understanding ties back to the scripture, emphasizing the importance of fermented foods. As omnivores, we require our foods to be more easily digestible. Fermented foods not only preserve the ingredients but also enhance digestibility. The fermentation process even mimics stomach acid, making the food easier for our bodies to break down and digest.

CHAPTER 21: FEVERS, THE LUNG/LARGE INTESTINE AND THE BIOFIELD

In Luke 4:38-39, it says that Jesus arose from the synagogue and entered Simon's house. Simon's mother-in-law was suffering from a high fever, and they asked him to help her. He stood over her, rebuked the fever, and it left her. Immediately, she got up and began to serve them (KJV).

There are interesting principles here. We often hear about how the Savior healed people through touch. However, I notice something significant regarding fevers and patients. Typically, fevers indicate that the large intestine is overly acidic. When this happens, the body can only push out toxins and inflammation through the skin.

We've previously discussed this in relation to the man with leprosy, but it also applies to fevers. When there is excess heat or inflammation in the colon that cannot be properly expelled, the body pushes it out through the skin. In this instance, the Savior did not need to touch Simon's mother-in-law; he simply stood over her.

I imagine he was within 5 or 6 feet from her body. Earlier, we mentioned the concept of the biofield—the energy field surrounding each person that typically extends about 5 or 6 feet from the body. When Jesus was in her proximity, he was within her biofield, affecting her energy system.

When he rebuked the fever, I believe he must have spoken with his voice, which activates the lung-large intestine power lines. This suggests that the woman had an issue related to this power line. The remarkable part is that simply by being nearby and speaking, he was able to help her overcome the fever.

Moreover, after her recovery, it's notable that she immediately stood up and began to serve. Even a small amount of movement can stimulate the lymphatic system, helping the body eliminate toxins and inflammation for a faster recovery.

CHAPTER 22: SUNSETS

In Luke 4:40, it is stated that when the sun was setting, people brought their sick to the Savior, who laid his hands on them and healed them (KJV).

We've discussed how the Savior's healing power is often associated with His touch, and it's interesting to note that people were brought to Him at sunset. Sunsets can be very healing for several reasons.

First, when you observe a sunset, you are treated to a spectrum of colors—typically red, orange, yellow, pink, blue, purple, and sometimes green. The variety of colors aid in the visual stimulus that contributes to emotional well-being.

Additionally, watching sunsets is beneficial for your body's circadian rhythm. Today, many spend less time outdoors, particularly during sunset. This lack of exposure can lead to difficulty falling asleep and feeling restless at night. Observing a sunset helps reset your circadian rhythm, making it easier to fall asleep. I learned this principle from Lois Lanee, one of my favorite experts on cranial nerves.

I've noticed this impact with my own children. If they use screens or watch movies after sunset, they tend to become overstimulated and find it hard to settle down for sleep. This overstimulation can lead to increased unhappiness as well. A simple way to help children (and adults) sleep better is to encourage them to go outside and watch the sunset.

Experiencing the full spectrum of colors can positively affect various energy pathways in the body. For example, the colors you see during sunset correspond to specific organs:

- Red can support the liver and gallbladder

- Orange can benefit the kidneys and bladder,

- Yellow relates to the spleen, stomach, and pancreas,

- Blue connects to the lungs and large intestine,

- Purple resonates with the sympathetic and parasympathetic nervous systems, and

- Green, though less common, aligns with the heart and small intestine.

- Pink, interestingly, goes with the heart, small intestine, liver, and gallbladder.

Thus, sunsets can engage and support all of these power lines. I encourage you to take some time to enjoy a sunset, as it not only helps improve your sleep but also contributes to your overall health and healing.

CHAPTER 23: MOVING WATER

In John 4:10-14, there are two references to living water. In verse 10, living waters are mentioned, and the Savior states in John 4:14 that "the water that I shall give him shall be in him a well of water springing up into everlasting life (KJV)." This illustrates the principle that moving water is healthy water.

We can observe this in nature. Stagnant water, which is not moving, tends to be diseased, often attracting mosquitoes and generally unhealthy. In contrast, moving water is clear, healthy, and more drinkable. One reason for this is that moving water creates a frequency. In rivers and creeks, the winding flow resembles the way frequencies oscillate, allowing for various healing principles.

One effect of moving water is the sound it produces. For instance, waterfalls generate frequencies ranging from 5 to 408 Hertz (Bedard, 2021; Boeckle, 2009). This frequency range resonates with the brain's theta, alpha, beta, and gamma waves, as well as impacting the liver and bladder power lines. Being near waterfalls can be healing, and the frequency of water that cascades over rocks contributes to this effect. As water moves over stones, it creates a charge; rocks have their own frequency that interacts with the water.

Thus, moving water is indeed healthy water. I appreciate the analogy the Savior provides because all movement and freedom come from Him. He created this earth, and all healing originates through Him. This idea is symbolic of our lives. When we are in motion and making progress, we don't have to be perfect; we simply need to try our best. There will be bumps along the way, but as long as we continue to move forward, He will always bless us—both spiritually and physically.

CHAPTER 24: HEALING AT A DISTANCE

In John 4:46-53, we read about a nobleman who came to the Savior because his son was seriously ill and close to death. Jesus told him, "Except ye see signs and wonders, ye will not believe." The nobleman responded, "Sir, come down ere my child die." Jesus said to him, "Go thy way; thy son liveth" The man believed the word that Jesus had spoken to him and went on his way (KJV).

Later, one of his servants met the nobleman and told him his son lives. The nobleman then inquired about the exact hour when his son began to heal. The servant replied, it was the seventh hour. At that moment, the nobleman realized that it was the same hour when Jesus had spoken to him, and he believed, along with everyone in his household (KJV).

The principle I gather from this story is the remarkable fact that healing can take place from a distance. When I think of distant healing, prayer is the first thing that comes to mind. When I was very sick and close to death I received prayers from many people, even those in different states, and I felt an immense sense of gratitude. Had it not been for those prayers, I honestly believe I wouldn't have made it.

Prayer is an incredible principle, and what's fascinating is that there are no limits on the distance from which healing prayers can be offered. When people pray for others, it not only empowers themselves but also brings strength to those for whom they pray. When multiple people pray for one individual, we witness the principle of resonance; all those prayers resonate and bring healing or comfort to the person in need.

We are also fortunate to live in a modern era. During COVID, the world changed significantly, and rather than meeting people in person, we found ways to connect from a distance. It's amazing what can be accomplished through simple nerve tests and patient histories on a telehealth call. Therefore, the principle of healing at a distance applies not only to prayer but also to modern technology, which offers the gift of healing to many people around the world.

Ultimately, all healing at a distance today is rooted in the Savior, Jesus Christ. He was the first to demonstrate healing from afar, and all the healing that occurs today is possible because of Him.

CHAPTER 25: OINTMENT, THE FEET, KISSING, AND THE HAIR AS AN ANTENNA

In Luke 7: 37-38, it describes a woman who had sinned who learned that Jesus was dining at a house. She brought an alabaster box of ointment and stood behind Him, weeping. She began to wash His feet with her tears, wiped them with the hair of her head, kissed His feet, and anointed them with the ointment (KJV). There are several important healing principles highlighted in this passage.

First, Jesus ultimately forgives this woman, demonstrating that He is the ultimate source of forgiveness for sin. Through Him, as we repent, we can receive forgiveness. However, there are also significant healing aspects in her actions.

Let's start with the ointment she brought. This ointment was likely a natural substance, as artificial products did not exist in those times. Whatever its chemical composition, it must have had healing properties. By applying it to Jesus's feet, she was benefiting from its natural healing properties by both smelling and touching the ointment.

The feet are powerful points for applying oils. There are multiple power lines that run through the feet, corresponding to organs such as the liver, bladder, kidneys, stomach, spleen, and pancreas. By applying the ointment to the Savior's feet, it enhanced His power.

While she wept and washed His feet with her tears, it's important to note that tears can be healing for various reasons. Holding back emotions is unhealthy, and crying is a natural way for our bodies to release those emotions. Additionally, producing tears activates the parasympathetic nervous system, which is responsible for our "rest and digest" functions. In this way, her weeping was beneficial not only for herself but also transferred healing energy to Jesus.

Another interesting detail is that tears are salty, and we will explore the significance of salt later. She wiped Jesus's feet with the hair of her head, which is also significant.

In 1 Corinthians 11:15, it says that if a woman has long hair, it is a glory to her (KJV). This phrase carries significant meaning, highlighting the power of hair.

Hair acts like an antenna for the body, a belief shared by some Native Americans I've spoken with. One individual shared that many Native Americans during World War II had to cut their hair to serve in the military. After cutting their hair, they noticed a decline in their ability to track objects. This suggests that the hair on our heads functions similarly to an antenna that receives frequencies.

In my experience working with patients who have suffered head traumas, concussions, or car accidents, I have observed that many men grow beards. This may serve as the body's way of enhancing proprioception. For women, however, long hair is especially powerful because it also functions like an antenna that transmits frequency. Through this act, she was infusing Jesus with additional power.

When she kissed His feet, she exhibited profound humility. Considering the hygiene practices of that time, their feet were likely very dirty. Kissing His feet represented not only her humility but also had physiological benefits. The act of kissing stimulates the trigeminal nerve (cranial nerve 5), one of the largest nerves in the body that conducts a significant amount of electrical signals. Kissing also causes the lips to come together, activating facial muscles and stimulating the facial nerve (cranial nerve 7), which is another parasympathetic nerve involved in resting and digesting.

Kissing His feet was not just a humble gesture; it was also a means of transmitting frequency from her body to His. The nerve pathways that connect various organs to the brain also run through the feet, making her kiss a powerful connection. Furthermore, a significant percentage of nerves in the body lead to the head. Thus, the woman kissing His feet served as a frequency donor for the Savior.

Ultimately, while her actions were significant, it is Jesus who possesses the ultimate healing power. By kissing His feet, she also created a channel through which He could heal her emotionally, alleviating the pain caused by her past sins.

CHAPTER 26: WE ARE NEVER ALONE

In John 4:7-9, we read, "There cometh a woman of Samaria to draw water. Jesus saith unto her, 'Give me to drink.' (For his disciples were gone away into the city to buy meat.) Then saith the woman of Samaria unto him, 'How is it that thou, being a Jew, asketh drink of me, which am a woman of Samaria? For the Jews have no dealings with the Samaritans (KJV).'"

This passage is particularly interesting because of the context in which the woman approached the Savior. In verse 6, we learn that this encounter took place at the sixth hour. We can interpret the sixth hour as having a digital root of 3, which symbolizes a time of healing (KJV).

It's important to note that this woman was a Samaritan, and during that time, Samaritans were looked down upon by Jews. This experience resonates with many of us today, as numerous individuals face labels imposed by others. These polarizing topics often lead people to separate themselves from one another, contributing to feelings of isolation.

The sense of isolation became especially common during COVID-19. Many people experienced significant mental discouragement and emotional pain due to isolation, whether it was enforced by laws and regulations or self-imposed.

I feel fortunate that my family and I lived in areas where we could remain active and connected with others, unlike some of my patients who struggled with the effects of isolation.

Additionally, technology and media can contribute to loneliness, acting as tools that lead to self-isolation. One of the crucial needs for our well-being is genuine human connection. When we are around others, there is an exchange of energy and frequency that is vital for our emotional and physical growth.

Ultimately, I want to emphasize that you are never alone. The Savior, Jesus Christ, knows who you are and is always there to reach out to you. He often uses others as instruments in His hands—sometimes in the form of unseen angels whose presence we can feel, and at other times through the support of other people.

In times of need, the Lord will send people to help you feel less isolated. So, if you ever find yourself feeling alone, grieving, or isolated, remember to turn to the Savior. He is always there to rescue and support you.

CHAPTER 27: LIGHT

In John 3:19-21, it states: "And this is the condemnation, that light is come into the world, and men loved darkness rather than light, because their deeds were evil. For everyone that doeth evil hateth the light; neither cometh to the light, lest his deeds should be reproved. But he that doeth truth cometh to the light, that his deeds may be made manifest, that they are wrought in God (KJV)."

This passage speaks about light and darkness, which is often a metaphor for spirituality. When we turn to the Savior, we are embracing the light, while choosing to follow the adversary leads us into darkness. Those who come to the Savior love the light.

However, this concept extends beyond spiritual truths; it also applies to the physical realm. Light has healing properties, as demonstrated by sunlight. Sunlight is one of the most healing elements, and I believe that the sun's healing capabilities symbolize Jesus Christ. It is no coincidence that The Savior is "The Son", and "sun", as in sunlight sound similar, and both are healing.

Unfortunately, in recent years, sunlight has been blamed for various illnesses, particularly skin conditions such as cancer. In reality, around half of skin cancer patients have low vitamin D levels, which is essential for numerous biological processes in the body

(Lombardo et al., 2021). Sunlight helps our bodies produce vitamin D.

Moreover, light in various forms can be healing, all of which can be seen as symbolic of the Savior. One type of healing light I like to use is red light. Red light therapy is effective for inflammation and pain relief, penetrating deep into the bones when at the correct wavelength. Another beneficial type of light is yellow light, which I find excellent for improving skin tone. As we age, our skin tone can diminish, but yellow light therapy helps to tighten the skin.

Green light is also effective; I have observed that it aids with weight loss in many patients. UV light, which can be described as a bright blue and purple light, is also healing. UV light must be the right wavelength and can help correct scarring, just like red light.

The body contains fascia, which functions like power lines. After surgery or trauma, the fascia can separate but the body reconnects the fascia with time, but often there is no power flowing through the area of the scar. Using specific light therapies like red, infrared, UV, and scalar in conjunction with essential oils can help restore this flow of power to the body.

Additionally, I have found that UV light is effective against various infections. I have treated patients with skin infections or shingles outbreaks that did not respond to other treatments, but when UV light is applied to the affected area, healing occurs more rapidly. Remarkably, viruses and bacteria cannot adapt to UV light; it is antimicrobial and effectively eliminates toxins and microbes.

In summary, light possesses healing properties, and once you discover and apply these principles, it can benefit not only patients but also individuals and their families. It is essential to remember that light is healing because it symbolizes The Savior.

CHAPTER 28: THE MOUNTAINS, SCALAR FREQUENCY, AND ALTITUDE

In Matthew 5:1, it says that when the Savior saw the multitudes, He went up into a mountain, and when He was set, His disciples came unto Him (KJV).

It's no coincidence that the Savior often chose to go to the mountains, especially considering His 40 days in the wilderness, which likely included mountainous regions. Mountains have always been regarded as holy places. For instance, the Lord appeared to Moses on a mountain.

There are several reasons for this. First, drawing closer to God often requires effort and action. When the prophets, and especially the Savior, went to the mountains, it was a demonstration of work and faith.

Another reason is that mountains have a pyramid shape, classified as a Platonic solid. In geometry, certain shapes can concentrate more frequency from the sun, specifically scalar frequency. When you are in the mountains, you are surrounded by this scalar frequency.

Additionally, altitude sickness is a well-known phenomenon associated with high elevations, but the body also adapts to these conditions over time. One important factor in this adaptation is red blood cells that contain hemoglobin, the protein in red blood cells that carries oxygen throughout the body. Research shows that spending at least two weeks in the mountains can alter your red blood cells, providing benefits that can last for weeks or even months and increasing your oxygen efficiency (D'Alessandro et al., 2016).

Oxygen is crucial because neurological function, especially in the brain, relies on three key components: glucose, frequency, and oxygen.

Thus, when the Savior ascended the mountains, He was continuing a tradition observed in scripture where prophets sought out these holy places. Not only is this practice spiritually enriching, but it also has significant benefits for both the body and the mind.

CHAPTER 29: SALT

In Matthew 5:13, it says, "Ye are the salt of the earth. But if the salt have lost his savour, wherewith shall it be salted? It is thenceforth good for nothing (KJV)." This verse introduces an interesting principle about salt.

Unfortunately, in our day, salt has often been portrayed as a negative substance, typically blamed for raising blood pressure. However, from what I've observed, the quality of the salt is what truly matters. Many modern salts not only lack good quality but we are also not consuming enough overall. This raises the question—why would the Savior use an analogy involving something that is considered bad? In fact, when it's of the right quality and quantity, salt can be good for you.

So, why is salt beneficial?

First, our bodies require power, and the more conductors we have, the better the power flows. Salt is an excellent conductor of power in the body. Considering the significant amount of liquid in our bodies, we need a good conductor for frequencies to flow through it.

Second, salt plays a crucial role in stomach acid production. Without sufficient stomach acid, our bodies struggle to function properly. Stomach acid is essential for digesting proteins—molecules made up of amino acids. When you have enough stomach acid, it helps break down proteins into amino acids, which are the absorbable building blocks of cells.

Additionally, the flavor of salt is vital. The cranial nerve 7, also known as the facial nerve, allows us to taste salt. This nerve is part of the parasympathetic nervous system, which helps the body with sleep, rest, and digestion.

I appreciate the analogy the Savior provides because salt is truly healing. Unfortunately, many modern salts have lost their beneficial properties due to being demineralized. Many companies have removed essential minerals from salt for other uses, resulting in products that aren't pure. Furthermore, some salts have various flavorings or preservatives added, including anti-caking agents like bromide, which is toxic and disrupts thyroid function and numerous biological processes.

My most trusted brand of salt is Redmond Real Salt. Through frequency and vibrational testing, I've found it to be the most beneficial for thousands of patients. If you're looking for a good quality salt, consider Redmond Real Salt.

Salt also serves as a natural preservative. It is commonly used in the pickling and fermentation processes, such as sauerkraut or kimchi. When foods are naturally fermented, not only are they preserved, but their probiotic content increases as well. Probiotics are essential for health, helping to fight infections and support digestion.

What's fascinating about this analogy is that the Savior is referring to us as well. I first heard this concept from Elder José A. Teixeira of the Presidency of the Seventy of The Church of Jesus Christ of Latter-day Saints. Just as salt is made of sodium and chloride, we can think of ourselves as one part, and the Savior as the other. When we bind ourselves to Him, we receive the most benefit and can positively impact those around us (Teixeira, 2024).

Salt helps us break down proteins, similar to how, when we are united with the Savior, we can assist in breaking down difficult situations. Salt also activates the parasympathetic system, which aids in digestion and promotes restful sleep. When we are connected to the Savior, we have the capacity to bring peace to the world around us.

Ultimately, all these healing principles stem from Jesus Christ. When we are bound to the Savior, we can act as preservatives for goodness in a world that has strayed spiritually.

I personally enjoy adding salt to each meal and even adding a dash to my water, as many of us are deficient. The Savior would never mention anything harmful to the body; rather, He highlights what is good. That's why salt is so powerful.

CHAPTER 30: HOW TO HANDLE YOUR ENEMIES

In Matthew 5:44, it says, "Love your enemies, bless them that curse you, do good to them that hate you, and pray for them which despitefully use you, and persecute you (KJV)."

This principle is especially important today because, from a health perspective, contention does not come from the Lord; it comes from the adversary. The reason the adversary thrives on contention is that it creates chaos. The human body does not function properly in chaos; it operates best with organization, harmony, and peace.

When we face attacks, whether verbal or otherwise, our natural human reaction might be to respond in anger. However, the Savior teaches us that every situation has its opposite. Instead of responding with malice towards an enemy, we can choose forgiveness, which resonates at a higher frequency. By loving, we adhere to a higher law that benefits our well-being.

If someone curses you, you can choose to bless them. This blessing can manifest in your thoughts, words, or through prayer. When you do good to those who persecute you, you are again embracing this higher law. Although applying these principles is not always easy, it is worth it.

I remember an experience from middle school when someone was unkind to me because of my beliefs. Instead of arguing back or retaliating, I decided to take the high road by being kind to them. Eventually, that person became a friend, even when others were not kind to them. I have seen the power of this principle frequently throughout my life.

It is essential to understand that our bodies are not meant for contention. I have often observed how disharmony and anger can lead to health issues.

By fostering more harmony and happiness and applying the Savior's principles of love, blessing others, praying for them, doing good, and serving others, you will increase your happiness.

Of course, there are times when we need to set boundaries, especially if someone is harming us or our families. You can still establish these boundaries while applying these principles. If you do, you will find yourself happier, healthier, and more successful in life.

CHAPTER 31: STRETCHING

In Luke 6:6-10, we read about the Savior in a synagogue on the Sabbath, where He interacts with a man who has a withered hand. The scribes and Pharisees are questioning whether He will heal this man on the Sabbath. In verse 10, we see the Savior telling the man to stretch forth his hand, and when he does, his hand is made whole, just like the other one (KJV).

An important principle here is that when the Savior asks someone to perform an action and they comply, it demonstrates their faith and willingness to act. By stretching forth his hand, the man was not only expressing his faith, but he was also engaging in a powerful physical principle.

Stretching has significant benefits; it activates the nervous system and increases power in the body. Furthermore, our fascia system functions like the power lines of the body, connecting different organs and constantly channeling frequency. You can also boost the power of the nervous system through stretching.

This is why practices like yoga, Pilates, and general stretching are so therapeutic: they ultimately enhance the frequency and vibration throughout the body.

Interestingly, in my work with athletes, I've observed that many prefer to stretch before their practices, workouts, or games. However, I believe this can be counterproductive. Stretching a cold muscle is like stretching a cold rubber band; it may not yield the best results. Instead, stretching should ideally occur after warming up the muscles. This approach can improve flexibility, enhance power within the system, and also help reduce the risk of injuries.

CHAPTER 32: VIRTUE WENT OUT OF HIM

In Luke 6:19, it states that the whole multitude sought to touch the Savior, and virtue went out of Him, and He healed them all (KJV). This concept is intriguing not only for healers but also for family members and caregivers.

As a chiropractor, I have observed this phenomenon in my practice. When I work on individuals, whether through massage or adjustments, I often feel drained afterward. This occurs because when I touch someone who is sick or injured, they have decreased power. In this interaction, I unintentionally transfer some of my power to help them heal, much like the Savior did.

The Savior, being the greatest healer of all, experienced this transfer of power Himself. If it happened to Him, it can happen to all healers. I've also noticed this in parents, especially mothers, who care for a sick child. They often feel drained as their energy is directed toward nurturing and healing their child.

This transfer of power occurs from a state of high power to a state of low power. Therefore, if you are a provider, practitioner, or caregiver, it's essential to find ways to replenish your own energy after taking care of someone else. There are various methods to do this. Sometimes, it's beneficial to pay for someone to help you, whether through massage, adjustments, or other treatments.

Other ways to restore your energy include exercise, grounding, or spending time in sunlight. It's crucial to engage in practices that help you regain your power. Throughout the scriptures, there are instances where people assisted the Savior, and He graciously accepted their help. If He, the greatest healer with unmatched power, needed support, then we, being less than Him, certainly need it as well.

CHAPTER 33: LOOKING UP

In Luke 6:20, it says that the Savior lifted up His eyes toward His disciples and said, "Blessed be ye poor: for yours is the kingdom of God (KJV)."

When we think about the Savior, we see He had immense compassion and mercy. He recognizes His disciples as being poor.

The term "poor" can have multiple meanings. Sometimes we may feel poor in spirit, in physical resources, or in health. When we find ourselves in such circumstances, it often triggers a sympathetic response—putting us in a fight-or-flight mode or creating stress.

However, one of the remarkable things about the Savior is that, instead of absorbing that same energy, He chose to lift up His eyes. There is something powerful in the act of looking up.

One way looking up helps us is through the eye muscles, which are controlled by something called cranial nerve III. This nerve activates most of the eye muscles. When we look up, cranial nerve III is engaged, which is a part of the parasympathetic nervous system that helps our bodies rest and digest.

So, when we find ourselves in stressful situations—whether they involve ourselves or others—try looking up. This simple action can help activate the parasympathetic system, allowing us to enter a more peaceful and calm state.

Ultimately, when we are in a state of rest and digest, we tend to make better decisions regarding our lives, health, and finances. This aligns with the Savior's message of having faith instead of fear.

CHAPTER 34: LAUGHTER

In Luke 6:21, it says, "Blessed are ye that hunger now: for ye shall be filled. Blessed are ye that weep now, for ye shall laugh (KJV)."

Laughter is essential for our health, yet it has significantly decreased in recent years. When COVID-19 began and people started wearing face masks, one major consequence was the reduction of laughter. This is because when you can't see someone smile or laugh, it diminishes your own ability to do so, which can negatively impact your well-being.

Laughter has several health benefits. First, it produces a frequency that typically ranges from 126 Hertz to 502 Hertz (Szameitat et al., 2011). This frequency can help alleviate pain and inflammation, as well as resonate with important power lines in the body, such as those related to the liver, kidney, and bladder. That's why laughing can sometimes give you the urge to use the bathroom; you're activating these power lines.

Moreover, when you laugh, you engage your facial muscles, which are stimulated by the facial nerve, also known as cranial nerve VII. This nerve is part of the parasympathetic nervous system, which helps your body relax and digest properly. Therefore, laughter activates these beneficial pathways and supports your body in overcoming sadness and sorrow.

It's crucial to prioritize laughter in our lives. It's unfortunate that much of today's comedy doesn't match the uplifting nature it used to have. While I fully support comedy, it should promote positivity and not harm others or yourself. There are countless things in life that can bring amusement, and that's something our society is missing right now. Finding humor is one of the best therapeutic practices we can adopt. So, get out there and embrace laughter!

CHAPTER 35: HAVING JOY AND LEAPING FROM OPPOSITION

In Luke 6:22-23, the Savior says that when people hate you, separate from you, or cast your name out as evil for the Son of Man's sake, you should rejoice in that day and leap for joy (KJV).

When we stand up for the Savior and defend Him, He promises blessings in return. There's a reason He encourages us to leap for joy when faced with opposition. Jumping or leaping increases your body's energy. I once attended a Tony Robbins event, and experienced an enormous boost in energy from jumping numerous times.

Opposition from others often leads to feelings of fear about what others might think. This fear can impact our bladder and kidney power lines. What I learned from Dr. Max Collins, is that when you jump and land on your heels, you activate a power line that starts from the bottom of your feet, goes through your heels, travels up the back of your legs and thighs, and extends all the way up your back to your head, including your cerebellum and occipital lobe.

Jumping and landing on your heels can help you overcome the fear of judgment from others. That's why the Savior instructs us to leap for joy in response to rejection; it not only helps us conquer our fears but also increases our body's power.

Again, the body is piezoelectric. Meaning when we move and exercise, we increase our body's power. The more power you have, the less you are affected by the negative energy of others.

CHAPTER 36: THE EYES AND LIGHT

In Matthew 6:22, it says that "the light of the body is the eye: if therefore thine eye be single, thy whole body shall be full of light (KJV)."

I appreciate this principle that the Savior teaches us, as He revealed knowledge that humanity had overlooked for centuries. Initially, people believed that the eye did not emit light, but recent research suggests otherwise—it indicates that the eye can emit light (Wang et al., 2011).

This is a powerful principle. It helps us understand that our eyes play a dual role: they both emit light and receive it.

This concept is important because, in today's world, we often see people wearing sunglasses. While sunglasses can protect our eyes from excessive sunlight, they also have drawbacks.

When our eyes look around, they can perceive different colors, which resonate with various frequencies in our bodies. For instance, when we gaze at green grass, the color green resonates with the heart and small intestine. Other colors, such as purple, resonate with the sympathetic and parasympathetic nervous systems. When we go outside and see these colors, they benefit our bodies and enhance our well-being.

However, wearing sunglasses can block the light that our eyes emit to others. It's disheartening to see so many people wearing sunglasses constantly. I remember walking one day and noticing that almost everyone I passed was wearing them. Not only did they appear sad, but I felt a sense of sorrow as well.

When we are able to make eye contact, it allows us to share our inner light with others. If we are thinking positive and loving thoughts towards people, we can radiate a beneficial frequency to those in need. If more individuals understood these principles and engaged with one another eye-to-eye, everyone would benefit.

Another modern challenge is the prevalence of phones and screens, which can be used for both positive and negative purposes. A downside is that when we look down at our devices, we stop emitting our light to the world and to others through our eyes.

So, I challenge you, instead of wearing sunglasses or staring at your phone while out in public, try to make eye contact with others. Let them feel your love and your light.

CHAPTER 37: WHAT TO EAT, DRINK, OR WEAR

Matthew 6:25-26 says:

"Therefore I say unto you, Take no thought for your life, what ye shall eat, or what ye shall drink; nor yet for your body, what ye shall put on. Is not the life more than meat, and the body than raiment? Behold the fowls of the air: for they sow not, neither do they reap, nor gather into barns. Yet your heavenly Father feedeth them. Are ye not much better than they (KJV)?"

Sometimes, when it comes to life and health, we can focus too much on what we're going to eat and what we're going to wear. I really like this scripture because it reminds us that the Lord observes the birds, which don't sow for food, nor reap, nor gather into barns, yet He feeds them.

Interestingly, when we look at birds, we can see what makes them healthy. For instance, I researched sparrows and found that they produce several frequencies with their pitch. These frequencies include 4521 Hertz, 4593 Hertz, 4608 Hertz, 4629 Hertz, 4758 Hertz, 6072 Hertz, and 6180 Hertz (Heij & Verboom, 2021). Remarkably, when you analyze these numbers, you'll notice they all add up to a digital root of 3, considered healing frequencies.

One of the things that contribute to the health of birds is their vocalizations or the frequencies they produce. Additionally, when birds fly and move around, they are exercising. I've observed this principle in my own life. During times when I've been sedentary, I tend to feel hungrier, but when I'm active and outdoors, I often feel more energized and don't need as much food.

We can learn from this scripture that sometimes we become overly focused on food and clothing when it comes to health. However, movement is essential, as is using our voice.

The Savior continues in Matthew 6:28, stating, "Why take ye thought for raiment? Consider the lilies of the field, how they grow; they toil not, neither do they spin (KJV)." Here, the Savior is addressing clothing. While it's important for us to wear modest clothing, as a society, I feel we don't get enough sunlight.

When we think about our ancestors and the amount of sunlight they received compared to us, it's clear that we live in structures that often confine us: our homes, cars, and workplaces. This limited exposure to sunlight can negatively impact our health. Therefore, spending time outdoors is crucial—not just for sunshine, but also for exposure to the various healing frequencies that nature provides. By simply embracing the principle of going outside, we can promote our growth, much like the lilies of the field.

CHAPTER 38: HOMES AND GNASHING OF TEETH

In Matthew 8:5-13, it is written that a centurion approached the Lord. In verse six, he explains that his servant lies at home, sick with palsy and suffering greatly.

Jesus responded, "I will come and heal him."

The centurion replied, "Lord, I am not worthy that thou shouldest come under my roof: but speak the word only, and my servant shall be healed. For I am a man under authority, having soldiers under me: and I say unto this man, 'Go,' and he goeth; and to another, 'Come,' and he cometh; and to my servant, 'Do this,' and he doeth it (KJV)."

This passage illustrates an interesting principle. The centurion felt unworthy to have the Savior enter his home. Our homes and workplaces can serve as places of healing or, conversely, can become environments filled with negative energy, depending on what is happening within them.

When we strive to choose light, keep the commandments to the best of our ability, and follow God, our surroundings can be filled with healing light. However, when there is negativity or harmful situations present, those spaces do not become places of healing. The centurion recognized this, and the Savior did as well.

In Matthew 8:13, Jesus said, "Go thy way; and as thou hast believed, so be it done unto thee (KJV)." And his servant was healed at that very hour. This showcases how, in my view, the Savior not only heals the servant suffering from paralysis but also has the power to heal our homes and environments.

Anytime I move into a new home, I always say a prayer for our family, asking that it becomes a safe place where the spirit can dwell and that it may serve as a healing space. I encourage everyone to do the same, not only for their homes but also for their workplaces or any places they spend the most time. You can transform wherever you are into a space of healing where the spirit can dwell through maintaining light in your life and surroundings.

An interesting verse is found in Matthew 8:12, where the Savior mentions that "the children of the kingdom shall be cast out into outer darkness: there shall be weeping and gnashing of teeth (KJV)." The term "gnashing of teeth" evokes the image of clenching or grinding one's teeth, which I often observe in our society. Many patients show signs of this, particularly in their temporalis muscles—the muscles located on the sides of the head above the ears that help close the jaw.

I have noticed that patients who are chronically stressed exhibit tightness in these muscles and tend to grind their teeth. This grinding will overstimulate the trigeminal nerve, also known as cranial nerve 5, which can drain considerable energy from the body. Additionally, when the teeth are clenched and grinding occurs, it results in sympathetic dominance, placing the body in a fight-or-flight response, which raises cortisol to unhealthy levels.

The body is designed for a state of rest and digestion, so finding ways to help the body relax and alleviate teeth grinding can make a significant difference. Many patients report a reduction in headaches and an overall sense of relaxation when they stop grinding their teeth.

There are various exercises to help with this, as well as new methods in biological dentistry designed to reduce teeth clenching and grinding, particularly at night. The comparison the Savior makes between outer darkness and gnashing of teeth is profound, as grinding negatively impacts physical health.

CHAPTER 39: TOUCHING THE HAND AND THE LARGE INTESTINE POWER LINE

In Matthew 8:14-15, it states that Jesus came to Peter's house and saw his mother-in-law lying sick with a fever. He touched her hand, the fever left her, and she got up and began to serve them (KJV).

It's interesting to note that the Savior touched her hand. Various parts of the body contribute to regulating body temperature, including the nerves and adrenal glands. In my personal belief, the large intestine also plays a significant role. When the colon becomes overly acidic, the body can eliminate illness and inflammation through the skin, often resulting in fevers.

The power line connected to the large intestine extends to the hand. By touching her hand, the Savior activated that power line and also stimulated the homunculus in the brain. A larger percentage of the nerves that connect to the brain originate from the face, hands, and feet.

What's remarkable is that not only did she recover, but after getting up, she began to minister to them. When individuals heal and then take action, it helps their bodies maintain the movement and energy necessary to assist not only themselves but others as well.

CHAPTER 40: PILLOWS AND THE FREQUENCY OF THE SPINE

In Matthew 8:19-20, it mentions that a scribe approached Jesus, expressing his desire to follow Him wherever He went. In verse 20, Jesus responds by saying, "The Son of man hath not where to lay his head (KJV)."

In my personal opinion, there are certain beneficial sleeping positions, and back sleepers should actually avoid using a pillow altogether.

If you are a side sleeper, using a pillow that maintains proper alignment is acceptable. A pillow can push your head forward, which places you in what I refer to as "adrenal phase." When your head is pushed forward, you enter fight-or-flight mode, making it difficult for your body to achieve restful sleep.

One reason I believe the Savior mentioned His lack of a definite resting place is that sleeping without a pillow can actually be healthier for back sleepers. Additionally, when the head moves forward, it reduces the natural curvature of the neck. The cervical spine is designed to have a slight curve, known as lordosis, with the apex of the curve at the front of the neck and a bend backward.

Today, however, many people have lost this natural curvature due to factors such as pillows, mouth breathing, excessive phone and computer use, and an inactive lifestyle. Interestingly, I think the shape of the spine can be viewed as a frequency. This frequency has various curves; it begins in the neck, peaks in the thoracic spine, and then descends again in the lumbar spine, which has a curve similar to that of the neck.

If we can maintain the proper frequency of our spinal structure, it can contribute to better physical health and increased vitality.

CHAPTER 41: RECOVERY, DEATH, AND SLEEP IN THE SHIP

In Matthew 8:21-22 it says that one of Jesus' disciples said unto the Lord, "suffer me first to go and bury my father. But Jesus said unto him, Follow me; and let the dead bury their dead (KJV)."

Even though this is a book about healing, this verse holds significant importance. It's crucial to recognize the Father's will, which we may not always understand. While the Savior had the power to bring the disciple's father back to life, He did not do so, likely because it was in accordance with the Father's will for that person to pass on.

In life, we often wish for the Savior to heal every ailment and prevent death. However, this is not always possible. We must learn to accept the Lord's will and timing, for His plan is perfect. When the Lord does heal and save, we should acknowledge His hand in those miracles.

Some of the most remarkable individuals I know, both young and old, have passed away. I believe that, in His mercy, the Lord sometimes takes these wonderful people home early to spare them from the sorrows and pains of mortal life. Those in the healthcare field need to recognize this as well.

When I first graduated and began working with many seriously ill patients, I hoped with all my heart that each of them would recover. But sometimes, we must accept the Lord's will and serve as instruments in His hands, doing our best to help others heal. We must trust that when we do everything we can, the Lord will take care of the rest.

The chapter continues in Matthew 8:23-24: "And when he was entered into a ship, his disciples followed him. And, behold, there arose a great tempest in the sea, insomuch that the ship was covered with the waves: but he was asleep (KJV)."

From this, we learn two important principles. First, the greatest healer of all, the Savior Jesus Christ, also needed sleep. Sleep is something we're often deprived of in our modern lives, especially those of us in healing professions. There comes a time when we need to care for ourselves and our bodies, just as the Savior needed rest.

Additionally, the Savior likely fell asleep for a reason. When you consider a ship, the rocking motion created by the waves can actually help one to relax and enter sleep mode. I learned about this phenomenon from Lois Lanee, a nerve expert. One effective technique that our ancestors used before falling asleep was rocking back and forth in a rocking chair, which isn't as common today. Rocking chairs helped reset the body at night.

This resetting occurs because of the action of the cranial sacral pump, which is located in your head and tailbone. This pump moves back and forth in a rhythm similar to a heartbeat, helping to flush toxins and inflammation out of the brain and spinal cord while bringing nutrients in. This movement also indicates that the parasympathetic system is engaged.

One technique I've used to assess whether someone is in a sympathetic (stressed) or parasympathetic (relaxed) state is the sway test. When individuals sway side to side, it indicates sympathetic dominance, whereas swaying front to back suggests a parasympathetic state. This rocking motion, whether from a rocking chair or the movement of a boat, aids in this resetting process.

It's no wonder the Savior was able to fall asleep amidst a storm, as His body experienced the calming, restorative motion of the waves, activating the cranial sacral pump to help him endure even in turbulent times.

CHAPTER 42: THUNDER

In Mark 3:17, when referring to his apostles James and John, the Savior calls them the "sons of thunder (KJV)."

When we think of thunder, we often associate it with something destructive. However, thunder also has interesting frequency principles. Typically, when there's thunder, there is lightning, which deposits power into the Earth's surface, soil, and dirt. While thunder itself doesn't strike the ground, we can hear it when it occurs.

The frequency produced by thunder is usually below 250 Hertz, with an average frequency around 63 Hertz (Abegunawardana et al., 2014). This particular frequency range resonates with vibrations that can help alleviate pain and also aligns with gamma waves in the brain. Research has shown that gamma waves are beneficial for healing—they assist with conditions like Alzheimer's and memory issues, as well as reducing inflammation and pain (Adaikkan et al, 2019; Martorell et al, 2019).

What's inspiring about this principle is that as followers of Jesus Christ, when we embrace and teach His principles, we not only experience personal healing but also have the ability to heal others.

This is why I find it meaningful that the Savior referred to James and John as the "sons of thunder (KJV)."

CHAPTER 43: PLANTING SEEDS

In Mark 4:3-8, the Savior tells the parable of a sower who went out to sow seeds. A sower is someone who plants seeds, and this parable discusses the different types of ground where the seeds landed. Most of these locations did not support growth, except for the seeds that fell on good ground, which produced plants yielding thirtyfold, sixtyfold, and even a hundredfold (KJV).

There is an important reason the Savior shares this parable. Throughout the earth, certain areas are known as energy gridlines, which intersect at right angles. Some of these grid lines have negative energy, where bad things can happen, leading to natural decomposition. Interestingly, ants, which rely heavily on decomposed food, will often build their mounds near or directly on these gridlines. Spiders likewise tend to weave their webs in these areas.

While these negative energy spots exist, there are also positive energy spots in nature. For instance, dogs often choose to lie down and rest in these beneficial areas. Birds can be observed circling above these good energy spots in the sky. When animals like dogs, wolves, or other canines are sick or injured, they instinctively seek out these positive energy locations to lay down and recover.

Understanding these principles highlights the presence of both good and bad energy areas, which can apply to gardening and farming as well. As someone who plants seeds or tends to gardens, it's beneficial to select good energy spots for planting.

In addition to identifying areas to avoid, you can also utilize the physics of shape to mitigate harmful energy spots, making them more conducive to plant growth. This knowledge is valuable in our time, and it's significant that the Savior was a master healer and understood the concepts of frequency and physics. We can apply these principles in our gardening techniques.

Another point worth mentioning is the digital root of 3. Notice that two of the numbers the Savior referenced in the parable—30 and 60—also have a digital root of 3. This connection is not random; it reflects a pattern that the Lord has established in the universe.

CHAPTER 44: MUSTARD SEED - SALVADORA PERSICA

In Mark 4:30-32, we read about the Savior comparing the Kingdom of God to a mustard seed. He described it as a small seed, but in verse 32, He noted that when it is sown, it becomes greater than all the herbs (KJV). He also mentioned that the birds of the air may lodge under its shade.

When people hear "mustard seed," they might think of the condiment that is used for hamburgers or hot dogs, which comes from the mustard plant in the Brassicaceae family. However, the mustard seed that the Savior referred to actually comes from a tree known as Salvadora persica.

Salvadora persica is a powerful herb known for multiple health benefits. It has antimicrobial properties, including antifungal, antibacterial, and antiviral effects, and it is also effective in fighting inflammation. Additionally, the herb contains monoterpenes (Elmhalli et al., 2019). This helps it resonate with the stomach, spleen, and pancreas.

This herb is important not only for those organs but also supports the thyroid, adrenal glands, and breast tissue in women. It is particularly beneficial for oral health and can help combat Porphyromonas gingivalis (Uddin & Kanatas, 2014). This is a microbial toxin that many patients with Alzheimer's or dementia symptoms are sensitive to.

This underscores why the Savior referred to mustard as one of the greatest herbs. As mentioned, birds tend to gather around beneficial energy spots, and the shade provided by this plant serves as protection from the sun and contributes positive energy. This powerful herb, often overlooked, is utilized in certain parts of the world, and there is a reason the Savior deemed it one of the greatest.

CHAPTER 45: FAITH CONQUERS FEAR

In Mark 4: 38-40, there is an account of the Savior sleeping on a boat during a great storm. The disciples, frightened by the tempest, woke him, saying, "Master, carest thou not that we perish?" In verse 39, we read that the Savior arose, rebuked the wind, and said to the sea, "Peace, be still." Instantly, the wind ceased, and there was a great calm (KJV).

Following this miraculous event, the Savior asked them, "Why are ye so fearful? How is it that ye have no faith (KJV)?"

I love how the Savior's response illustrates both his power and the lesson for us. He has the power to overcome all challenges, including great storms. This story serves as a testament to his ability to calm our fears. It also teaches us an important lesson about handling stress in our lives, whether those challenges are within our control or not.

Often, when faced with difficulties, people tend to panic. This panic can lead to sympathetic dominance, which usually results in poor decision-making. The disciples were panicking, but when the Savior arose to rebuke the sea, he was able to calm the storm because he remained calm himself. This serves as a reminder to turn to Him during life's storms and, no matter what we face, to remain calm and trust in Him. Everything will ultimately work out. I also appreciate that he questioned them about their fear: "Why are ye so fearful? How is it that ye have no faith (KJV)?" This highlights the concept of polarity, where every emotion has an opposite. For instance, fear affects the kidney and bladder power lines. When fear dominates our lives, it will decrease the power in the kidney and bladder so that they will not function like they should.

The opposite of fear is faith. By cultivating faith—not just thinking about it but also expressing it through our words and actions—we can overcome any fear we encounter in our lives.

CHAPTER 46: WOOD

In Luke 7:12-15, we find an account that takes place at night by the city gates, where a dead man is being carried out. When the Lord saw the grieving mother, He was moved with compassion. He approached and touched the bier, which is the stand that holds the casket. He said, "Young man, I say unto thee, Arise (KJV)."

After this, the dead man sat up and began to speak, and Jesus delivered him back to his mother. This passage presents several important principles. First, the Savior demonstrated His power through His voice, using it to raise the dead. Additionally, the act of touching the bier is significant. Previously, Jesus had healed people from a distance as well as by touching them directly. However, in this instance, He chose to touch the bier itself.

I imagine that the bier was made of wood, which, although it does not conduct electricity, still possesses its own vibrations and frequencies. When we look at wood, we notice its growth rings often form a pattern known as the Fibonacci sequence—this pattern is observed throughout nature, down to the level of DNA.

Even though wood is not a conductor of electricity, it still allows some form of vibration and frequency to flow through it. This phenomenon is also evident in nature; for instance, when lightning strikes, it can travel through wood. Lightning itself carries frequency and power, demonstrating that the Savior's power could flow through the wood of the bier into the deceased man to help raise him from the dead.

Ultimately, the Savior holds all power. However, what I take from this principle is applicable to our modern lives: we should consider using more natural materials in our homes and furniture. Many of the items we encounter today are synthetic, whereas our ancestors relied on natural materials like wood. While wood may not conduct electricity, it still carries vibrations that can contribute to a healthier living environment compared to synthetic alternatives.

CHAPTER 47: CO-SLEEPING

In Luke 11:5-8, the Savior presents a parable, asking, "Which of you shall have a friend, and shall go unto him at midnight, and say unto him, Friend, lend me three loaves (KJV)." The mention of the number three is significant, as it frequently appears in scripture. The parable continues, noting that a friend has come to visit and is in need.

In verse 7, it states, "And he from within shall answer and say, 'Trouble me not: the door is now shut, and my children are with me in bed; I cannot rise and give thee.'" However, verse 8 emphasizes a key point: "I say unto you, Though he will not rise and give him, because he is his friend, yet because of his importunity he will rise and give him as many as he needeth (KJV)."

We should also note the timing of this event, which occurs at midnight. Midnight, the 12th hour, also has a digital root of three. When considering the concept of a friend in this context, especially as it relates to the Savior, we recognize the friendship as a profound one. The mention of children being in bed brings to mind the concept of co-sleeping.

Co-sleeping is often frowned upon in modern Western culture, especially for young babies. However, opinions on this can vary greatly among parents. I remember when my wife and I brought our oldest child home. We had a crib ready, but she struggled to sleep in it. I recall my first night as a father, where I barely managed one or two hours of sleep due to her restlessness. However, when my wife began nursing her in our bed, she slept much better, perhaps only waking once for feeding.

Co-sleeping changed our lives, allowing both the baby and us to get a better night's sleep. I believe this is partly because our bodies emit a biofield that extends around six feet. Children can recognize their parents' biofields, and when a baby is placed in a crib away from their parent, they may feel a sense of danger or loneliness, which disrupts their sleep. In contrast, when co-sleeping, the baby can feel the presence of their parents, both through physical touch and this biofield, allowing for more deep sleep.

While co-sleeping might not suit every family, one principle I've noted is that mothers tend to be lighter sleepers than fathers. This seems to stem from mothers' innate feeding intuition, particularly regarding the needs of their newborns, for whom breast milk is the best option. Because mothers are lighter sleepers, it's generally safe for them to co-sleep with their babies. On the other hand, fathers tend to be deeper sleepers, making it essential to take precautions while co-sleeping.

In our experience, when my wife needs to nurse, I position myself lower in the bed, with my head at about the baby's waist. This way, my baby can sleep beside us while I can sleep deeply without the worry of rolling over onto them. There are also various safety attachments designed to make co-sleeping safer.

As for the question of when children should stop co-sleeping with their parents, this varies according to individual families and their specific needs. I've observed that even older children may desire to sleep in their parents' bed at night, which is perfectly normal. It's ultimately a matter of each family deciding when the time is right. In my view, co-sleeping should not be looked down upon, as typically happens in Western culture.

The principles of co-sleeping have not only been beneficial for my family but have also positively impacted thousands of families worldwide, who share similar experiences.

CHAPTER 48: GRIEF AND BLUE WATER

In Matthew 14:12-13, we read about the death of John the Baptist, who was related to Jesus Christ. Verse 12 states that John's disciples took his body, buried it, and then went to inform Jesus. In verse 13, we see that when Jesus heard the news, he departed by ship to a desolate place (KJV).

John the Baptist held significant importance to Jesus; he baptized Jesus and was part of his family. Losing someone you love, especially a family member, brings about feelings of grief. Jesus experienced this kind of sorrow for John.

Notice that Jesus chose to go to a desolate place by ship. While there were other routes he could have taken on foot to reach nearby deserts, he opted for a journey over water. This choice matters because water is known to have healing properties. The waves of the ocean often follow a Fibonacci pattern, which is associated with healing frequencies. Additionally, the color of water is blue, and in my experience working with patients dealing with grief, I've found that the color blue can be very beneficial.

The color blue resonates with the lung and large intestine in ancient Ayurvedic medicine, commonly known as the throat chakra. By being on the ship and looking at the blue water, it likely provided Jesus with some relief from his grief.

Another important lesson from how Jesus processed his grief is that it's okay to seek solitude to grieve and take a break from others. However, we also see in verse 14 that when Jesus saw the large crowd following him, he was filled with compassion for them and healed the sick.

Even in our moments of grief or difficulty, there is always someone suffering more than we are. By serving others, we cultivate gratitude, which is healing in itself. Just as Jesus served others despite his own sorrow, we, too, can find solace in acts of service during our grief.

These insights can be valuable for anyone mourning the loss of a loved one or facing challenging times—using the color blue, being around water, allowing ourselves space to grieve, and serving others can help us heal, just as it helped The Savior.

CHAPTER 49: GMO'S AND HEIRLOOM SEEDS

In Matthew 15:13, The Savior says, "Every plant, which my heavenly Father hath not planted, shall be rooted up (KJV)."

One of the insights we can draw from this scripture is that it speaks not only to the past but also to our present day. When the Savior mentioned that every tree or plant not planted by the Heavenly Father would be rooted up, it can be related to heirloom seeds. Heirloom seeds are original, time-tested seeds that have remained viable for generations.

The greatest scientist of all is God, who created this world and everything in it perfectly, because He is perfect. Unfortunately, in our time, humanity has attempted to uproot what God has created. One of the most significant examples of this is the use of genetically modified organisms (GMOs) or GMO seeds.

Many people believe their scientifically developed seeds are superior, but in reality, the seeds that God originally created are the best. I have observed this in the health of my patients. Many of them are gluten-free or gluten intolerant, yet quite a few can handle what I consider to be heirloom seeds or heirloom breads, such as kamut.

Kamut has been around for thousands of years and is an heirloom seed. Based on my observations, even gluten-intolerant patients can usually tolerate kamut flour, particularly when it is used in sourdough bread. Sourdough fermentation breaks down the gluten, making it more digestible.

I believe it is a significant mistake for humanity to think they can create something better than what God has made. God has provided everything we need on this earth—every seed, every plant, every animal, and even the smallest insects—down to the finest details, all for our use and benefit.

By trusting in Him and everything He has provided us, our bodies can truly thrive.

CHAPTER 50: WORDS, COMMUNICATION, AND POSITIVITY

In Matthew 15:17-18, it is stated that you may not understand that whatever enters the mouth goes into the belly and is cast out into the draught. Verse 18 says, "But those things which proceed out of the mouth come forth from the heart; and they defile the man (KJV)." Our words hold significant power; they can be used for both good and bad.

Several other scriptures expand on this idea. Ephesians 4:29 advises, "Let no corrupt communication proceed out of your mouth, but that which is good to the use of edifying, that it may minister grace unto the hearers (KJV)." This principle applies not only to how we speak to others but also to ourselves.

Philippians 2:14 instructs us to "do all things without murmurings and disputings (KJV)." This applies to life in general, to business, and also to our health. Furthermore, in Colossians 3:8, we are told to "put off all these; anger, wrath, malice, blasphemy, and filthy communication out of your mouth (KJV)."

When we examine these scriptures on the power of words, it becomes clear that they are emphasized for a reason. The Lord desires us to use positive and uplifting words. This applies not just to ourselves but also to how we speak about others. Unfortunately, in our culture today, it is common for people to use negative language.

This negativity can refer not only to inappropriate language but also to negative thoughts about ourselves or others. Hence, we should strive to maintain a positive outlook.

This reminds me of an experiment conducted by Dr. Masaru Emoto. He studied water in detail and performed an experiment where he had people say negative things to water, or played bad music near it, which resulted in the water becoming disorganized and murky. Conversely, when he had people pray over the water or express positive thoughts about it, or when he played uplifting music, the water became crystalline and organized (Emoto, 2004).

Given that a significant percentage of our bodies is water, the positive things we say about ourselves and others can help elevate our body's vibrations. This organization down to the cellular and microscopic level, such as with water, leads to higher frequencies and better electron flow.

This concept is important not only for ourselves but also in relation to others. Sadly, our age is filled with hate and anger, both in-person and, especially, online. By speaking positively about others, we can not only uplift ourselves but also contribute to their healing.

For those who work with patients, maintaining a positive dialogue about them—both in their presence and away from them—can significantly aid in their healing process. This change begins with our thoughts. By looking to our Savior Jesus Christ and reaching out for help through prayer, we can begin to shift our mindset.

It is also important to consider the media we consume. For example, I do not have a television, as I notice that many TV shows and movies are filled with negativity. When negativity is portrayed that way, it can affect our culture as a whole. This is why I prefer to read the Word of God, which is positive and uplifting.

Surrounding ourselves with positive and uplifting people will also help us maintain this outlook. I have found that the healthiest individuals I know are some of the most positive people, and they tend to be successful not just in their health but in life overall. No matter your current state, you can always make changes for the better. The quicker you start this process, the sooner you will notice improvements in your body, mind, and spirit.

CHAPTER 51: CLAY

In John 9:6, we read about a man who had been blind from birth and came to the Savior. When he approached Him, the Savior spat on the ground, made clay from the spittle, and anointed the blind man's eyes with the clay. Then He instructed him to go and wash in the pool of Siloam. The man obeyed, washed, and came back able to see (KJV).

There are several important principles to note in this healing event.

First, the clay used by the Savior is a material known for its healing properties. I have personally used bentonite clay for various reasons. I've consumed it to aid internal health, and applied it topically on my skin. I find clay to be very healing as it promotes circulation in tissues, facilitating the healing process.

Additionally, many people are unaware that our eyes have a microbiome, which consists of both good and bad bacteria. An imbalance, particularly an overgrowth of harmful bacteria, can lead to blindness. Clay acts as a prebiotic, helping to nourish and support the beneficial bacteria in both the eyes and the body at large. By placing clay on the blind man's eyes, the Savior was adding prebiotics that can enhance the microbiome.

Moreover, clay serves as a powerful binder. It binds to toxins such as heavy metals, chemicals, and microbial toxins that can be harmful. By doing this, clay helps to eliminate these harmful substances while simultaneously promoting a healthy microbiome.

Clay also originates from the soil, which possesses its own unique frequency. When the Savior applied the clay to the blind man's eyes, it improved the microbiome, bound to toxins, and increased the power of the eyes. This process was activated by the saliva of the Savior; any time we introduce saliva or moisture into the body, it has an additional aspect of healing.

The eyes particularly require lubrication, and dry eyes can contribute to blindness. By using both clay and saliva, circulation and moisture to the eyes were improved, also aiding in healing. And when the blind man washed in the pool, we know that water serves as a cleansing agent.

These principles can certainly be applied to overall body care, but clay, in particular, stands out as one of the most remarkable healing materials available. Many patients have experienced significant benefits from it as well. My favorite type of clay is bentonite clay, the top quality brand being Redmond clay. Regardless of the type of bentonite clay you choose, it's essential to follow the usage directions, as it has numerous applications for both internal and external health. It's truly an amazing healing material.

CHAPTER 52: LIGHT, CRANIAL NERVE 3, BALANCE, MASKS, AND LAZARUS

In John 11:9, Jesus states, "Are there not twelve hours in the day? If any man walk in the day, he stumbleth not, because he seeth the light of this world (KJV)."

It's interesting that He mentions there are 12 hours in the day, as the number 12 often appears in scripture and is related to the digital root of 3. This concept underscores the power of being outdoors during daylight. Waking up just before sunrise allows you to witness the beautiful colors of the dawn, which can enhance the functioning of various organs in our body.

Being in sunlight during the day also provides the significant benefit of vitamin D. When exposed to sunlight, our bodies produce this crucial vitamin, which is important for overall health.

Additionally, exposure to sunlight helps our eyes adapt to light. To do this, our pupils need to constrict, and this process is assisted by cranial nerve 3. This nerve is a part of the parasympathetic system and helps the body rest and digest. Furthermore, cranial nerve 3 controls most eye muscles, except for the lateral rectus and superior oblique muscles. Effective eye movement supports our balance, which is why Jesus said we "stumble not." When our eyes can accurately gauge our body's position in space, it enhances balance.

For patients struggling with balance issues, one of the best recommendations is to spend time outside, particularly in sunlight.

Finally, watching the sunset before bed also offers benefits. This experience provides varying frequencies of light and helps reset your circadian rhythm, making it easier to fall asleep and enjoy deeper rest.

For all these reasons, it's clear why the Savior spoke of the significance of the light of the day.

In John Chapter 11, we read about the death of Lazarus. In John 11:32-35, when Mary came where Jesus was, she fell at His feet and said, "Lord, if thou hadst been here, my brother had died." When Jesus saw her weeping, He was troubled, and it says that "Jesus wept (KJV)." This is a powerful scripture, as it shows that Jesus, the Son of God with all power, felt emotions just like we do. It's important to recognize that even the greatest healer of all time expressed His emotions, and this is a healthy way to respond to grief.

In some generations, showing emotion has been frowned upon, but this passage demonstrates that tears are not a bad thing. If the Lord Himself wept, then it's clear that tears can be healthy. When we cry, our parasympathetic nervous system is activated, which helps our bodies rest and digest. This response also prevents us from holding onto emotions that could negatively impact our health.

As the chapter continues, we see that they went to the grave. In John 11:39, Jesus said, "Take ye away the stone (KJV)." Martha, the sister of Lazarus, replied, "Lord, by this time he stinketh: for he hath been dead four days (KJV)." Jesus responded in John 11:40-41, "Said I not unto thee, that, if thou wouldest believe, thou shouldest see the glory of God (KJV)?"

"Then they took away the stone from the place where the dead was laid. And Jesus lifted up his eyes, and said, Father, I thank thee that thou hast heard me (KJV)."

There are several principles from this story that I appreciate. First, I want to acknowledge all the caretakers of those who are sick or injured. When I was younger and unwell, my parents made significant sacrifices for my care, both financially and emotionally. I believe the Lord has a special place in His heart for those who care for others.

During my recovery, I met a young woman who helped me tremendously. Despite my struggles, she remained kind and supportive while dating. Her patience and care for me were invaluable. That young woman became my wife, Ashley, and now we have built a wonderful life together.

This highlights the beauty of having people who care for you—family members and professionals in clinical settings such as hospitals, hospice, and funeral homes. These caretakers deserve great recognition. The Lord will bless those who sacrifice to help others. In my experience with patients, many cannot recover alone; they need their family's support. Just as I received help during my healing journey, Lazarus had support from his family.

Jesus could have rolled away the stone Himself, but He asked them to do it. It's interesting to note that Martha, Lazarus's sister, expressed discouragement, saying he had been dead for four days and that there was a smell. However, Jesus provided her with faith and hope. If you find yourself in a caretaker role, remember that there is always hope. Keep pressing forward, and the Lord will help you through your trials.

After they removed the stone, I find it significant that Jesus lifted His eyes and thanked the Father for hearing Him. He lifted His eyes in prayer rather than bowing His head, which is a common gesture of reverence. Lifting one's gaze can stimulate cranial nerve 3, which is part of the parasympathetic nervous system, promoting rest and digestion. Additionally, looking up at the bright sky causes the pupils to constrict, which is also run by cranial nerve 3. When this parasympathetic nerve is firing, it enhances the overall power of our body.

Later, we read in John 11:43 that Jesus "cried with a loud voice, Lazarus, come forth (KJV)." In John 11:44, it describes the miracle that followed, "and he that was dead came forth, bound hand and foot with graveclothes: and his face was bound about with a napkin. Jesus saith unto them, Loose him, and let him go (KJV).

There is a principle that I find important in this context. During the COVID pandemic, many people were required to wear face masks. From my experience seeing numerous patients, I noticed that these masks had a negative impact on many individuals. Personally, I experienced discomfort wearing a mask; it hurt my jaw and made it feel like I couldn't breathe. I observed that many of my patients struggled with the same issues.

It's one thing for people to choose to wear masks for their own reasons, but it's quite another for them to be forced to do so. I believe in the importance of personal agency. For those who opted to wear masks during COVID, that was their choice. However, my personal belief is that no one should be mandated to wear them.

This reminds me of the passage where the Savior spoke about Lazarus, who was bound in great clothes on his hands, feet, and face. The Savior commanded in John 11:44, "Loose him, and let him go (KJV)." I think this principle is significant in our time. Just as the Savior had them free Lazarus so he could breathe, I believe that being able to breathe freely without a mask is essential for our well-being. Oxygen is vital for our nerves, hormones, and recovery.

While I may not have the power myself to raise someone from the dead like the Savior did, I have faith that if it is the Lord's will, people can be raised from the dead with the Lord's power. I've never had the opportunity to heal someone in that way, but I firmly believe in the power of our Savior, Jesus Christ, who is the greatest healer.

CHAPTER 53: THE TEMPLE, GOLD, CRYSTALS, STONES, PEARLS, AND LINEN

In Matthew 23:17, it states, "Ye fools and blind: for whether is greater, the gold, or the temple that sanctifieth the gold (KJV)?" This verse raises an important question regarding the concept of sanctification.

Sanctifying means to make something holy or pure. So, why would a temple, which serves as a sanctifier, make gold holy and clean? The answer lies in the nature and purpose of the temple itself.

The temple present during Jesus' time is known as Herod's Temple, which was constructed from limestone and marble (Harash, 2020). These materials enhance the gold's frequency and have a cleansing effect. This is not merely a spiritual principle but also has physical implications. Many ancient temples, including Herod's Temple, utilized what are called Platonic solids—certain geometric shapes that can help magnify frequency. Herod's Temple had a shape similar to a cube, which contributed to its ability to cleanse the gold.

Materials can absorb frequency, similar to how different colors and shapes absorb heat. The design of ancient temples was intentional:

it allowed them to absorb beneficial energy while blocking harmful energy. This leads to the question posed by the Savior: Is the gold itself greater than the temple that sanctifies it?

Other scriptures also reference gold, evidence of it being such a high vibration material including:

- Revelation 8:3, which mentions an angel having a golden censer, as well as incense, which would benefit Cranial Nerve 1.
- Revelation 14:14, which refers to a golden crown, symbolizing kingship and potentially enhancing brain function due to the crown's color and material.
- Revelation 21:15, which speaks of a golden reed (KJV).

Furthermore, in Luke 19:38-40, as the disciples proclaim, "Blessed be the King that cometh in the name of the Lord," some Pharisees ask Jesus to rebuke them. Jesus replies that if the disciples were silent, "the stones would immediately cry out (KJV)." This statement suggests that stones possess frequency as well.

Another reference to stones is found in Revelation 21:11, describing a light that resembles a "stone most precious, even like a jasper stone, clear as crystal (KJV)." It goes on to mention that the walls of this heavenly city are made from jasper and also discusses gold, concluding with the phrase "like unto clear glass (KJV)." This signifies that clear materials like glass can resist negative frequencies. Just as different colors can absorb heat, they can also absorb negative frequency, while clear materials do not.

Additionally, Revelation 21:19-20 lists various stones, including jasper, sapphire, emerald, and amethyst (KJV). This highlights the unique frequencies and vibrations of each one. These frequencies can positively impact not only the human body but also living environments. Some scholars have found that ancient acupuncturists used stones and crystals instead of needles (Ramey & Buell, 2004). For instance, even though shungite is not mentioned in the scriptures, research indicates that it can block harmful electromagnetic radiation (Kurotchenko et al., 2003). Thus, when the Lord mentions stones and crystals, it serves a purpose. Utilizing these materials not only harmonizes one's environment but also benefits the body.

Lastly, in 2 Timothy 2:20, it notes, "In a great house there are not only vessels of gold and of silver, but also of wood and of earth (KJV)." This inclusion of silver is significant. Silver is known for its high frequency and vibration; it can melt ice faster than other metals due to these properties and is recognized for its antimicrobial benefits. My favorite silver product is colloidal silver, which has proven antimicrobial properties (Vila Domínguez et al., 2020).

If you've ever heard the phrase "someone's been fed with a silver spoon," it's commonly used to describe someone who is wealthy. This term originates from the time of the bubonic plague when the wealthy would use silver spoons to feed the sick, believing that silver could help protect them (Mosher, 2022).

Colloidal silver is something I've personally used, along with my family and thousands of patients, and I've witnessed its remarkable effects.

Another material worth mentioning is wood. Woods contain alcohols, monoterpenes, and sesquiterpenes (*Oil chemistry wheel* 2018; *Using the Wood Essential Oils* 2025). These chemicals resonate with the lungs, large intestine kidneys, bladder, stomach, spleen, pancreas, and the sympathetic and parasympathetic nervous systems. This is why having wooden items in the home or the scent of wood can be so healthy and therapeutic.

Additionally, there's a special mention in the scriptures, particularly in Revelation 21:21, which states that there are 12 gates made of pearls, with each gate being a single pearl. It also notes that the streets of the city were made of pure gold that was as clear as glass (KJV). This ties back to the earlier themes of gold and transparent materials that do not absorb harmful frequencies.

An interesting fact about pearls is that within pearl oysters, there lives a fish that produces a frequency ranging from 100 to 1000 Hertz (Kéver et al., 2014). This frequency can help alleviate pain, reduce inflammation, and resonate with various vital areas in the body, including the liver, gallbladder, kidneys, bladder, spleen, stomach, pancreas, heart, small intestine, lung, and large intestine, as well as the sympathetic and parasympathetic nervous systems.

It's no wonder that women across different cultures are drawn to pearls. Wearing pearls is thought to promote strong feminine energy and healing due to both the frequency they emit and their physical properties. The natural shiny white color of pearls is significant as well; white hues are associated with shielding from harmful frequencies. Furthermore, pearls have a spherical shape, categorized as a platonic solid, which enhances their scalar frequencies.

Interestingly, though oysters are deep underwater and do not see sunlight, they still receive frequencies from ocean waves. These waves create a Fibonacci pattern, and additional frequencies can also come from marine life such as whales and dolphins.

Additionally, the depth of the ocean increases pressure which also enhances the frequencies. Thus, there are healing principles to be found both above and beneath the water.

Lastly, another important material is referenced in Revelation 15:6, which mentions the seven angels coming out of the temple, dressed in pure white linen and girded with golden sashes (KJV). This again points to gold, but the angels are clothed in pure white linen. White fabric is significant as it does not absorb nearly as much harmful energy from EMF or radiation, and linen itself carries a powerful frequency.

Research by Dr. Yellen found that linen has a frequency of about 5000 Hertz (Crawford-Yellen, 2013). From all the patients I have worked on, this frequency resonates with the vagus nerve, aiding in pain management, activating the vagus nerve, and alleviating stress. Therefore, wearing linen is another excellent choice for healthier clothing materials.

CHAPTER 54: HEARING, A SPEECH IMPEDIMENT, CRANIAL NERVES 8 AND 10

In Mark 7:32-35, we read about a man who was deaf and had a speech impediment, and people brought him to the Savior. In verse 33, it says that Jesus took the man aside from the crowd and put his fingers into his ears (KJV). By doing this, He was employing several principles, as He placed His fingers in both ears.

This act demonstrates the principle of frequency. One finger acts as a positive conduit, while the other functions as a negative one. By placing His fingers in both ears, He was completing an electrical circuit, much like bringing the north pole of a magnet close to the south pole—when they are opposite, they attract and complete the circuit, allowing for the flow of frequency.

The ears are significant as they house various nerve pathways, notably those connected to the gallbladder, which ties into our ability to hear. From a nerve perspective, two important nerves are involved: cranial nerve VIII (the vestibulocochlear nerve), which aids in hearing, and cranial nerve X (the vagus nerve), which we'll discuss further in a moment. By simply placing His fingers in the man's ears, the Savior was completing this circuit.

Then, in the next part, we read that He spat and touched the man's tongue. This action stimulated salivation, which activates the parasympathetic nervous system, known for its healing properties. The vagus nerve, which is cranial nerve X, plays a crucial role in this parasympathetic response.

Finally, in the next verse, the Savior looks up to heaven, sighs, and says, "Be opened." When He gazed upward, it likely caused His pupils to constrict. This constriction activates cranial nerve III (the oculomotor nerve), which is also part of the parasympathetic system. When activated, the parasympathetic system helps unlock the body's frequencies and power, enhancing overall well-being.

Moreover, the constriction of the pupils acts as a funnel for light, which is another source of healing energy that flows through the Savior's arms to facilitate healing in the deaf man. When He speaks the words "be opened," He is engaging another frequency aspect, as discussed earlier.

As a result of these combined actions—looking heavenward, speaking with intention, and activating the parasympathetic system—the Savior was able to enhance the power and frequency within the deaf man's body. What follows, as noted in verse 35, is that immediately, the man's ears were opened, and the string of his tongue was loosened, allowing him to speak plainly.

One reason he could speak again is that the vagus nerve (cranial nerve X) was activated, allowing the uvula and the palate to vibrate, as well as providing innervation to the tongue. The deaf man had what I refer to as a "tongue tie," which I often see in patients. When individuals experience tongue tie, they typically have a deficiency in cranial nerve X.

There is another scripture that relates to this idea of tongue tie. In Acts 2:26, it states, "Therefore did my heart rejoice, and my tongue was glad; moreover also my flesh shall rest in hope (KJV)." One reason the heart rejoices is that a grateful tongue can express joy. The ability of the tongue to rise is crucial; many people with tongue issues struggle to breathe properly because they cannot elevate their tongues to the roof of their mouths.

As mentioned in my second book, the proper positioning of the tongue is essential. Ideally, the tongue should press against the top of the mouth, akin to a dolphin arching its back. Difficulty in raising the tongue can lead to signs of tongue tie and airway issues. These airway complications can hinder the body's healing process.

When the tongue is able to move upward, it stimulates cranial nerve X—the vagus nerve—which, in turn, supports heart function. This is why the scripture states that the heart will rejoice, and it highlights the significance of our physical and emotional well-being. We learn that the parasympathetic system aids us in resting, relaxing, and digesting, helping us navigate stressful situations with hope.

One of the most powerful things you can do is to position your tongue toward the roof of your mouth or suck it upward like a dolphin, which can activate your parasympathetic nervous system, improve your breathing, and empower your body.

CHAPTER 55: SPIKENARD

In Mark 14:3, it says that while Jesus was in Bethany, at the house of Simon the leper, a woman came with an alabaster box of spikenard ointment, and she poured it on the Savior's head (KJV).

Interestingly, we've previously discussed leprosy, a condition characterized by skin issues. Based on my observations, leprosy often correlates with decreased power in the lungs and large intestine. It's no coincidence that spikenard oil was present in the house of a leper. This oil contains sesquiterpenes, which resonate with the kidneys, bladder, lungs, and the large intestine—key power lines in the body. The act of applying it to the Savior carries deeper significance.

When she applied the spikenard to Jesus, it symbolized His sacrifice. He suffered for all our sins and pains, and this woman's offering was a way to help balance those vital power lines, which are crucial for both physical and emotional well-being. Spikenard oil is also known to assist with emotions such as grief and fear.

The head is a powerful area for applying frequencies or essential oils, a fact that many people might not be aware of. Most of the body's major power lines pass through the head. Additionally, when considering the homunculus of the brain, a significant percentage of the nerves that connect to the brain come from the face, head, hands, and feet. Thus, this was an inspired choice by the woman to apply the oil in this manner.

I've found that some of the best healers are women, due to their strong intuition. This serves as a lesson for us all—while the Savior is the greatest healer, He too needed to be served. Understanding these principles of frequency and how they relate to our organ systems, along with which oils resonate with specific power lines, can help explain principles found in scripture and everyday life.

CHAPTER 56: SORROW AND HEALING THE HEART THROUGH THE SAVIOR, JOY, PRAYER, THE SCRIPTURES, AND SERVICE

In John 16:22, it says, "And ye now therefore have sorrow: but I will see you again, and your heart shall rejoice, and your joy no man taketh from you (KJV)."

When we experience traumatic events in life and feel sorrow, it corresponds with a lack of joy. These emotions can drain our heart's power. The opposite of sorrow, or a lack of joy, is rejoicing. This is one way to combat negative feelings and help raise the frequency of our hearts. It's important to remember that Jesus spoke these words to His apostles, who knew He would eventually die but also that He would be resurrected. By looking to the Savior, we can also find reasons to rejoice.

I appreciate that the scripture emphasizes that no man can take joy from us. Too often, we depend on others for our emotional state in today's culture, and we feel sorrow because of negativity from others about ourselves. However, the Lord intends for us to thrive independently. We can rely on our Savior, Jesus Christ, to always find joy.

In Luke 24:17, The Savior said to the apostles, "What manner of communications are these that ye have one to another, as ye walk, and are sad (KJV)?" Here, the Savior addressed the sadness of His disciples following His death. Later, in Luke 24:25, He points out, "O fools, and slow of heart to believe all that the prophets have spoken (KJV)." This shows that sadness can diminish the power of the heart.

After the apostles realized it was the Savior, they later said in Luke 24:32, "Did not our heart burn within us, while he talked with us by the way, and while he opened to us the scriptures (KJV)?" Their sadness affected their hearts, but when they were in the presence of the Savior, they felt the Spirit, which ignited a burning feeling within them. This burning sensation is one manifestation of the Spirit, emphasizing that the Spirit brings healing.

Communicating with the Savior through prayer and engaging with the Scriptures can help alleviate feelings of sorrow or a lack of joy. These practices uplift our hearts. When we study the Scriptures, we invite healing into our lives.

Lastly, in 2 Corinthians 9:7, it says, "Every man according as he purposeth in his heart, so let him give; not grudgingly, or of necessity: for God loveth a cheerful giver (KJV)." Another way to enhance the power of our hearts is through giving. This can mean donating material items or contributing our time.

There are many individuals around us who need help. Often, when we feel sorrow or a lack of joy, it's because we compare ourselves to others and feel inadequate. However, many people around us may be in more challenging situations. By serving others, practicing gratitude, and giving, we can feel God's love. When we give cheerfully, it also raises the power of our hearts, which is why I believe the Lord emphasized this.

CHAPTER 57: ALOE

In John 19:39, we read about Nicodemus who first came to Jesus at night, bringing a mixture of myrrh and aloes (KJV). We have already discussed myrrh, but aloe is particularly interesting. The aloe plant is known for its ability to thrive in the desert and is widely recognized for its skin-healing properties.

Upon further examination, we find that aloes contain phenolics (Bawankar et al., 2014). Phenolics help the heart and small intestine power lines. It is no wonder that aloe is also known to be beneficial for the gastrointestinal (GI) tract.

When I was seriously ill in the past and struggling with digestion, one of the things that provided relief was aloe vera gel and aloe vera juice. It was soothing to my GI tract, and now I understand that it was likely due to the phenolics it contains.

This serves as another sign of the Savior's healing capabilities. That's why Nicodemus brought it; the Savior is the ultimate healer, and all these natural remedies are just tools in His hands. Being the Creator of this earth, He has placed numerous healing materials around us, like aloe vera, which we can use not only to support our digestive health but also for the care of our skin.

CHAPTER 58: THE ATONEMENT OF JESUS CHRIST, OLIVE TREES, OLIVES, AND OLIVE OIL

In John 12:12-13, we read about the Savior's grand entry into Jerusalem, in which the people took palm branches to greet Him (KJV). This highlights important principles related to healing. This event took place before the Savior, Jesus Christ, performed His Atonement and faced crucifixion.

The act of greeting Him with palm branches is significant for a few reasons. First, it symbolizes the greeting of a king. Additionally, there's a health principle to consider: this occurred around Passover in the springtime, and most likely the palms they used were date palms. Date palms at that specific time produce a distinct aroma.

When the crowd waived these palm branches at the Savior, they released an aroma that filled the air. Notably, this aroma contains sesquiterpenes and phenolics (Elhefni et al., 2023). Sesquiterpenes are known to resonate with the lung and large intestine, while phenolics resonate with the heart and small intestine.

Interestingly, we learn from Isaiah 53:3-5 that the Savior would bear our griefs and sorrows (KJV). Grief is known to affect the lung and large intestine, while sorrow or a lack of joy impacts the heart and small intestine. Therefore, when the people greeted Him with the scent of palms, it supported and prepared Him to bear our sorrows and grief.

In Matthew 26:36-39, it describes how Jesus, along with His disciples, went to a place called Gethsemane. He instructed them to sit there while He went to pray, taking Peter, James, and John with Him. In Matthew 26:37, it says He began to feel sorrowful and very heavy. Then, in Matthew 26:38, Jesus expressed to His disciples, "My soul is exceeding sorrowful, even unto death: tarry ye here, and watch with me." In Matthew 26:39, He went a little further, fell on His face, and prayed, saying, "O my Father, if it be possible, let this cup pass from me: nevertheless not as I will, but as thou wilt (KJV)."

During this time, Jesus experienced what we refer to as the Atonement—when He suffered for the pains, sins, and sorrows of everyone who has ever lived. While I cannot fully comprehend the depth of His pain, it is significant that He chose Gethsemane for a specific reason.

The Garden of Gethsemane is filled with olive trees.

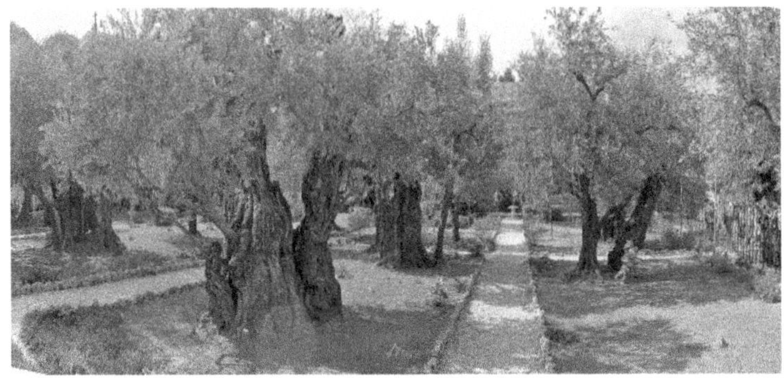

Image: "Old Olive trees in the Garden of Gethsemane" By Beko is licensed under CC BY 4.0

Olive trees serve as a powerful symbol. Olives are pressed to produce olive oil, known for its health benefits and healing properties. However, to create olive oil, olives must be squeezed and endure pressure—much like what the Savior experienced. He took upon Himself all the sins and pains of the world, and because of His suffering, we have the opportunity to overcome our own sins and pains through Him.

Interestingly, some of the olive trees in Gethsemane can live for an extremely long time. Being around trees can be healing; touching a tree can enhance our well-being. Additionally, trees create a toroidal field, similar to that of the human body, which may have provided some support to Jesus during His time of pain.

Olive oil contains phenols and alcohols (Zielińska et al., 2020). Phenols resonate with the heart and small intestine power lines. The sorrow Jesus felt indicates a lack of joy, and phenols can help alleviate that feeling.

Alcohols, on the other hand, can assist the parasympathetic and sympathetic nervous systems. When these systems are out of balance, it can lead to anxiety, placing the body in a fight-or-flight state dominated by cortisol and stress. Anyone undergoing such intense circumstances would experience this; however, as the Son of God, Jesus was capable of overcoming all things.

Being surrounded by the olive trees may have offered Him some physical, mental, and emotional support during this incredibly stressful time. Yet, it is crucial to understand that no one on earth, except Jesus Himself, has endured the pain He suffered. Because of His experience, we can find ways to overcome our troubles with His help.

This understanding gives special meaning to me whenever I use olive oil or eat olives. They remind me of our Savior, Jesus Christ, and serve as a symbol of His healing and support.

CHAPTER 59: VINEGAR AND THE VAGUS NERVE

In John 19:29, we read about the Savior while he was on the cross. It states that the Roman soldiers set a vessel full of vinegar, filled a sponge with vinegar, and put it upon hyssop, and put it to His mouth (KJV).

While we know that the Savior later died, he was resurrected on the third day. The act of giving him vinegar is interesting because the bitter taste activates cranial nerve 10, also known as the vagus nerve.

Vinegar is powerful for healing. One way we use vinegar is in the pickling process, where we preserve food naturally, making it more digestible. The bitter taste can stimulate cranial nerve 10, which I have used with thousands of patients, observing amazing benefits related to this vital nerve.

The vagus nerve is associated with the parasympathetic system, helping the body to rest and digest. What's remarkable is that vinegar's healing properties are symbolic of our Savior, Jesus Christ during his time on the cross.

So, if you want to activate your vagus nerve, incorporating bitter tastes like vinegar into your routine is an effective method.

CHAPTER 60: SCHUMANN RESONANCE, WHITE, AND SNOW

When the Savior, Jesus Christ, was resurrected, the description of His countenance in Matthew 28:3 states that His appearance was like lightning and His raiment, also known as clothing, was as white as snow (KJV). This raises an interesting principle: when we think of His countenance being like lightning, we can relate this to the frequency of lightning when it strikes the earth.

Lightning creates a phenomenon where electrons bounce back and forth between the ground and the atmosphere, resulting in what is known as the Schumann resonance. This resonance typically measures around 7.83 Hertz (Tang et al., 2019). This may explain why spending time outdoors with your bare feet in the grass or dirt can be healing.

Additionally, His raiment being described as "white as snow" is significant. The color white absorbs fewer harmful frequencies. When snow is examined under a microscope with detailed imaging, we can observe sacred geometry within its structure.

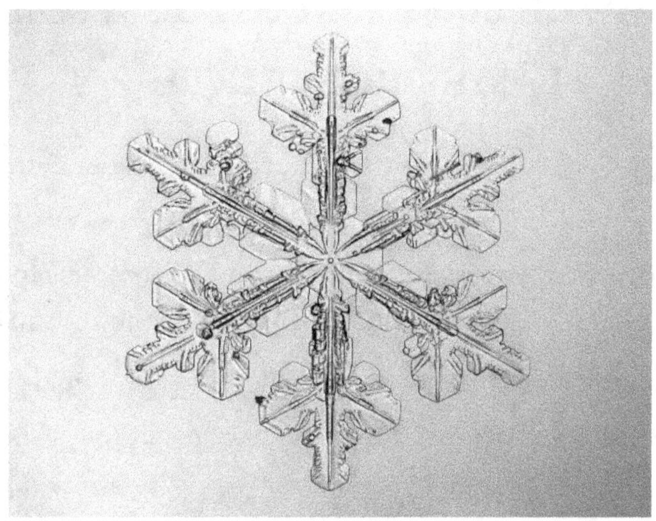

Image: "Snowflake (lumehelves)" By Janek Lass is licensed under CC BY 4.0

Most snowflakes have six points, which corresponds to the digital root of 3. This pattern of sacred geometry is found throughout the universe and represents a level of organization.

When water is structured, as seen in the case of snow, it has healing properties. It is remarkable that this description of the Savior reflects that everything about Him is inherently healing.

CHAPTER 61: PETER HEALS A MAN LAME FROM BIRTH

In Acts 3:6-7, after the Savior was crucified and resurrected, He bestowed power and authority upon Peter to lead His church. The scripture describes a man who was lame from birth coming to Peter during the ninth hour, which has a digital root of three. When the man asked for money, Peter responded, "Silver and gold have I none; but such as I have give I thee: In the name of Jesus Christ of Nazareth rise up and walk (KJV)." Peter then took the man by his right hand and lifted him up, and immediately the man's feet and ankle bones received strength (KJV). This passage marks one of the first instances of Peter using the power from the Savior to heal someone.

What is particularly fascinating is that when Peter took the man by the hand, he was connecting the power of the Savior to both the man's power lines through his fascia and nervous system. Our hands and feet connect to all the power lines of our body, but also a significant portion of our body's sensory input is processed in the brain, represented by the homunculus. Therefore, when Peter lifted the man, he enabled the flow of power from the Savior, allowing him to stand and gain strength instantly.

The next verse, Acts 3:8, states that the man "leaping up stood, and walked, and entered the temple, walking, and leaping, and praising God (KJV)." This reaction is remarkable; instead of cautiously walking for the first time, he chose to leap, which amplifies the power in the body. It is significant that he went to the temple immediately, as the temple serves as a place of healing, both physically and spiritually. When someone who has previously been unable to walk or leap regains their abilities, it often inspires a deep desire to serve God, which is evident in this man's choice to go to the temple.

CHAPTER 62: THE INVISIBLE THINGS OF HIM

In Romans 1:20, it states, "For the invisible things of him from the creation of the world are clearly seen, being understood by the things that are made, even his eternal power and Godhead; so that they are without excuse (KJV)."

One interpretation of the "invisible things" mentioned in this scripture is not only spiritual matters but also the principles of frequency.

While there are different wavelengths of light that our eyes can see, frequency itself is also something we cannot visibly perceive. We can hear it, and we can feel it—it's an invisible phenomenon.

Colossians 1:15-16 further emphasizes this by stating, "Who is the image of the invisible God," and in verse 16, "For by him were all things created, that are in heaven, and that are in the earth, visible and invisible, whether they be thrones, or dominions, or principalities, or powers: all things were created by him, and for him (KJV)." This highlights the significance of both the visible and invisible being created by Him, which includes frequencies.

Frequencies can manifest in various forms, including materials and sounds, as well as in specific locations. Throughout this book, we've also explored the concepts of power, emphasizing that all things were created by Him and for Him.

As you read this book, you will come to realize that all these principles of frequency, physics, power and healing ultimately point to the Savior, Jesus Christ, who is the creator of this earth.

This is why Philippians 2:10 states, "That at the name of Jesus every knee should bow, of things in heaven, and things in earth, and things under the earth (KJV)." This includes frequencies, which will work to our benefit when we draw closer to the Savior and strive to follow Him and adhere to His teachings.

By doing so, we can harness the power of frequency and healing to our advantage because of Him.

CHAPTER 63: FRUIT IN SEASONS, HUMIC AND FULVIC

In Acts 14:17, it says, "he did good, and gave us rain from heaven, and fruitful seasons, filling our hearts with food and gladness (KJV)." Here, "fruitful seasons" is a key concept. Many people don't realize that frequency has a timing aspect as well.

The Lord has everything planned out perfectly.

Fruits come into season for a specific reason. When we eat fruit in season, it aligns with its natural frequency, which resonates better with our bodies because the fruit is thriving. Eating fruit that is out of season doesn't benefit our bodies as much.

I'm not suggesting that you can't eat fruit outside of its season; however, consuming fruit in season provides the best benefits.

Additionally, in Revelation 22:2, it states that "in the midst of the street of it, and on either side of the river, was there the tree of life, which bare twelve manner of fruits, and yielded her fruit every month: and the leaves of the tree were for the healing of the nations (KJV)." There are several principles of frequency in this passage.

The mention of "twelve manner of fruits" is significant because the number 12 has a digital root of 3, a number associated with healing. Again, we see the principle of seasonality, as the tree yields fruit every month and its leaves are meant for healing.

Leaves need chlorophyll to undergo photosynthesis. In the fall, when the leaves fall, chlorophyll breaks down due to the microbiome of the soil, which naturally deposits nutrients back into the soil. Among these nutrients are humic and fulvic acids. Humic is a powerful nutrient that many soils now lack because they have been treated with fungicides.

Fungicides inactivate the mold and fungus that break down the leaves, leading to nutrient-depleted soils and, consequently, nutrient-depleted food. Humic and fulvic acids are essential for health; I have used them with thousands of patients and observed amazing results, particularly in detoxing. They also help balance minerals at the cellular level.

If there is one superfood that people are missing in their diets, it's humic. This is why it is said that "the leaves of the tree were for the healing of the nations (Revelation 22:2, KJV)."

CHAPTER 64: MASCULINE ENERGY AND INTIMACY

In 1 Corinthians 16:13, we are introduced to the concept of masculine energy, complementing our previous discussions about feminine energy. The verse states, "Watch ye, stand fast in the faith, quit you like men, be strong (KJV)."

Unfortunately, in today's culture, we are witnessing a trend of demasculinization often labeled as "toxic masculinity." In my opinion, this term is misleading and serves as a tool of the adversary to promote weakness in men. However, God desires strong masculine energy in men.

Exercise is one effective way to cultivate this strength. While we will discuss exercise in more detail later, it is crucial to recognize its importance. I believe that many distractions in life, often influenced by the adversary, prevent us from becoming our best selves. Our healthiest selves can be achieved through movement.

For men, in particular, having a desire to exercise is essential for cultivating masculine energy.

Regarding strength, 2 Corinthians 12:10 reminds us: "Therefore I take pleasure in infirmities, in reproaches, in necessities, in persecutions, in distresses for Christ's sake: for when I am weak, then am I strong (KJV)." This verse highlights that when we focus our strength on the Savior, we can find strength even in our moments of weakness. It's a principle that many overlook: God cares about every detail of our lives, including our strength. When we pray for increased strength or physical capabilities, we must also put in the effort through exercise.

While it's vital to strive for physical strength, balance is equally important. We can sometimes get overly focused on our bodies. Ephesians 5:28-29 states, "So ought men to love their wives as their own bodies. He that loveth his wife loveth himself. For no man ever yet hated his own flesh; but nourisheth and cherisheth it, even as the Lord the church (KJV)." One way to serve our bodies is by loving our spouses.

In our culture, many men struggle with negative self-talk, which is detrimental. We should practice loving ourselves by taking care of our physical health—eating well, exercising, and maintaining a positive mindset instead of tearing ourselves down.

Furthermore, Ephesians 5:33 states, "Nevertheless let every one of you in particular so love his wife even as himself; and the wife see that she reverence her husband (KJV)." This consistent theme of love is not just for ourselves and our relationship with God, but also for one another, especially between husbands and wives.

A common issue I observe among couples is fighting, which is often normalized in media. However, fighting and contention are not the Lord's way; they are the adversary's tactics. Instead, we should aim to love one another and handle conflicts in a way that reflects the Savior's teachings. This approach enhances our personal power and raises the positive energy in our homes, workplaces, and communities.

Lastly, Ephesians 5:31 teaches, "For this cause shall a man leave his father and mother, and shall be joined unto his wife, and they two shall be one flesh (KJV)." This profound statement underscores the importance of unity in marriage. I have seen relationships suffer when couples rely more on their parents instead of turning to God and each other. This can create significant challenges in both their relationship and their health.

When couples face difficulties, it's common for them to turn to their parents instead of seeking guidance from God or confiding in each other. This tendency can lead to marital issues because the couple may not address their challenges with the Lord or communicate openly with one another. Inviting God to help guide your marriage is a must.

Intimacy is a vital aspect of the concept of "one flesh." Unfortunately, many people have a distorted view of intimacy. However, when intimacy is practiced within the framework that God has established within the bonds of marriage, it can transform your life.

In my second book, "Biohacks of Intimacy", I focus on the physical dynamics. While there are spiritual, mental, and emotional dimensions of intimacy, my book covers the physical health dimensions of intimacy. I discuss concepts like biohacks and frequency principles that can enhance this aspect of a relationship. Intimacy is powerful—not only does it bring children into the world, but it also serves as a healing force within the bounds of marriage. When a man and a woman come together as one flesh, their feminine and masculine energies align, creating a connection similar to bringing the positive end of a magnet close to the negative end. This unity generates a powerful connection between both husband and wife.

Additionally, intimacy benefits the immune system and plays a role in resetting the autonomic nervous system. This reset can enhance parasympathetic function, promoting better rest and digestion. So if you are married, and you are struggling to have a satisfactory quality and quantity of intimacy with your spouse, there are solutions referenced in my book. Improving your intimacy will not only help you grow closer together but will also improve your health overall.

CHAPTER 65: HOW PARENTS SHOULD NURTURE THEIR CHILDREN

In Ephesians 6:4, it states that fathers should not provoke their children to wrath, but instead bring them up in the nurture and admonition of the Lord (KJV).

As we previously discussed, it is unhealthy for couples to fight with one another, not only for their mental, physical, and emotional well-being but also for that of their children.

Often, when we yell at our kids or say things that are not in harmony with the Savior, we cause harm. While we don't have to be perfect, what matters is that we strive to do our best. When we approach parenting with patience and love, we help our children's developing minds grow positively.

I have worked with many young patients, and unfortunately, a significant amount are under a great deal of stress. Part of this stress stems from social media, where they constantly compare themselves to others. This comparison is detrimental to their mental health, as they are often exposed to negativity online, in schools, and in various other situations. As a result, many children have lost the confidence they once had.

When children receive negativity from their own parents at home, it creates an environment that doesn't feel safe. The scripture reminds us to bring them up in nurture and admonition of the Lord. One principle that I suggest every parent follows in raising their kids positively is to be intentional. This approach helps give children the confidence and love they need.

Additionally, reading the scriptures with them or discussing examples of how the Savior would respond can be very beneficial. Christ loves all people, especially children, because of their innocence and capacity for love. The Savior encourages us to be childlike in our faith.

When we turn to Him and embody His love in our parenting, it benefits us and serves as a reminder of the power of children in our lives. If we engage with our children positively and speak to them with kindness, they will grow up to be a strong and incredible generation.

CHAPTER 66: GROUNDED

In Colossians 1:23, it says, "If ye continue in the faith grounded and settled, and be not moved away from the hope of the gospel, which ye have heard, and which was preached to every creature which is under heaven; whereof I Paul am made a minister (KJV)." The word "grounded" is significant here. It speaks to a spiritual perspective—when we are grounded in Christ, we become unshakeable.

This grounding is not only spiritual. There is also a physical aspect to it. For example, when we walk barefoot in the grass, dirt, or sand, we connect with the earth and draw energy into our bodies. This power comes from God's creation, specifically through Jesus Christ, who made this incredible earth with its remarkable healing properties. Thus, being grounded—both spiritually and physically—holds great power.

CHAPTER 67: COUNTERING CONTENTION WITH SALT

In Colossians 4:6, it says, "Let your speech be alway with grace, seasoned with salt, that ye may know how you ought to answer every man (KJV)." We often discuss the importance of avoiding conflicts and refraining from saying things we might regret. However, when we express positive thoughts, it elevates the frequency and vibration in our bodies. A fascinating biohack to consider is the use of salt.

Salt can be particularly beneficial in contentious situations. When we are in a contentious environment, our bodies can enter sympathetic mode, triggering the fight-or-flight response. In this state, we may feel compelled to argue or even withdraw, which increases the likelihood of saying something we would later regret.

To counteract this, we can activate the parasympathetic nervous system, which promotes relaxation. One effective way to do this is simply by tasting salt. If you find yourself about to enter a frustrating situation, such as a disagreement at home or any other conflict, try putting some salt in your mouth.

The reason this technique works is that the sensation of tasting salt involves cranial nerve VII, also known as the facial nerve, which is part of the parasympathetic nervous system. This nerve helps your body to relax and supports the "rest and digest" process. Thus, reducing your instinct to fight back. So if you ever feel the need to "throw down", then throw down that good quality salt on your taste buds and relax.

CHAPTER 68: NOT BEING WEARY IN WELL DOING

In 2 Thessalonians 3:13, it states, "But ye, brethren, be not weary in well doing (KJV)." This message is important in every aspect of life, whether it's school, work, or any other task we may face. Approaching these tasks with low energy can lead to negative consequences for our mental, physical, and emotional well-being.

When we go through the motions without enthusiasm, we can end up in a state of stress, choosing between fighting against or fleeing from our challenges. However, the scripture encourages us not to become weary in doing good. Even when obstacles arise, if we tackle them with energy and excitement, we can transform our experience.

Our energy and enthusiasm can be conveyed through the words we use and our body language. Engaging with life in this positive state not only makes our tasks more enjoyable but also helps us complete them more quickly. Furthermore, our positive energy can uplift those around us.

While it may seem simple, this approach is incredibly powerful and can be beneficial in our everyday lives and health.

CHAPTER 69: MARRIAGE, MEAT, AND ANIMALS

In 1 Timothy 4:1-3, it says "that in the latter times some shall depart from the faith, giving heed to seducing spirits, and doctrines of devils; Speaking lies in hypocrisy; having their conscience seared with a hot iron; Forbidding to marry, and commanding to abstain from meats, which God hath created to be received with thanksgiving of them which believe and know the truth (KJV)."

We must believe and embrace the truth, as 1 Timothy 4:4 states that "for every creature of God is good, and nothing to be refused, if it be received with thanksgiving (KJV).

This description resonates well with our current times. When discussing health, the issue of forbidding marriage is significant. Many might assume that healthier patients are often single since they have more time to focus on their well-being. However, I have consistently noticed that my married patients tend to be healthier. Marriage is a powerful institution, not just for individual health but also for our communities.

The family is the most basic unit of society. Strong families lead to strong communities, which in turn create strong cities. Strong cities contribute to strong states, and strong states build a strong nation. Ultimately, this foundational structure starts with the family, making marriage an important aspect.

Additionally, in our culture, there are movements aimed at eliminating meat consumption entirely. From my observations, the body typically requires at least a small amount of meat. Patients who completely abstain from meat often lack sufficient nutrients in their systems, as well as essential fats and proteins. Therefore, avoiding meat altogether can be detrimental to health.

There are other scriptures that mention meat as well. For instance, Hebrews 5:14 states, "but strong meat belongeth to them that are of full age (KJV)." Further references to meat can be found in Luke 7:37 and John 4:8.

When discussing thanksgiving, it is crucial to understand the need for moderation. In my personal opinion, patients who exclusively eat meat and neglect other foods tend to struggle with undigested proteins. We are intended to consume a variety of foods, including fruits and herbs, as God created all things on earth for wise purposes.

Moreover, our relationship with animals is not solely about consumption; being around them can also be healing. For instance, when animals are outside and active, their fur acts like an antenna for frequencies. Interacting with them increases our own energy. Additionally, animals, particularly dogs, produce sounds that are within a healing frequency range.

Therapeutic animals, like dogs and horses, are beneficial for many people. Horses, in particular, emit a variety of frequencies that can have healing effects. However, it is essential to engage with all of creation in a spirit of thanksgiving and wisdom.

While some may take dietary or lifestyle choices to extremes, it is important to acknowledge that God created animals for various purposes, including both consumption and companionship. All creatures contribute to our health and well-being.

CHAPTER 70: EFFECTIVE EXERCISE

In 1 Timothy 4:8, it states "bodily exercise profiteth little: but godliness is profitable unto all things, having promise of the life that now is, and of that which is to come (KJV)." I've discussed the importance of movement and exercise; however, I believe that moderation in all things is equally important.

When you engage in intense exercise for prolonged periods, it can lead to elevated cortisol levels in the body (Torres et al., 2021). Cortisol is known as the stress hormone. I often hear from patients who say, "I try to work out for one to two hours, but after my workout, I'm so tired that I can't do anything else the rest of the day." This is an example of over-exercising, where increased cortisol levels result in decreased testosterone (Khan et al., 2023). A drop in testosterone can hinder recovery and increase fatigue.

For middle-aged and older adults, exercise is best limited to a time frame of about 10-15 minutes. Teenagers can handle longer workouts, while young adults should aim for sessions not exceeding 30 minutes. One efficient method to maximize benefits is High-Intensity Interval Training (HIIT).

In HIIT, you perform an exercise intensely for 30 to 60 seconds, followed by a short rest, and repeat this for approximately 12 minutes. This approach is one of the best ways to boost testosterone, which is vital for energy and weight loss. Unfortunately, many people either don't exercise enough or end up overdoing it.

Incorporating biohacks can make your workouts more efficient, one being blood flow restriction bands. These bands allow you to achieve the equivalent of a one-hour workout in just 10 to 15 minutes. You can find these bands at https://healingplaybook.prob3.com/.

We are fortunate to live in a time where God has provided innovative techniques and technologies that help us maintain our health so that we can serve Him and others effectively.

1 Timothy 4:12 continues by saying, "Let no man despise thy youth; but be thou an example of the believers in word, in conversation, in charity, in spirit, in faith, in purity (KJV)." Many of these attributes are not only spiritual but also shape our mindset. Sadly, in today's world, particularly on social media, individuals often face backlash for striving to be their best selves. Those who engage in such attacks are often grappling with their own insecurities; in an effort to elevate themselves, they tend to bring others down.

However, it is vital to remember that God loves us unconditionally, and we do not need approval from others. What truly matters is pleasing God. When we strive to gain His trust and do our best to follow Him — spiritually, physically, mentally, and emotionally — we can become our healthiest selves. This enables us to help others who are in need.

CHAPTER 71: A LITTLE LIQUID

In 1 Timothy 5:23, it says to "drink no longer water, but use a little wine for thy stomach's sake and thine often infirmities (KJV)." I previously discussed alcohol consumption, and back in biblical times, wine was one of the few clean sources of liquid available.

Today, we have the convenience of access to clean drinking water, but I believe one of the key principles here is moderation in liquid consumption. I was first introduced to this idea by Dr. Max Collins, who pointed out that many people often drink too much liquid. In my experience with patients, excessive liquid intake can overwhelm the kidneys, preventing them from filtering effectively. This can lead to a condition known as water retention or excess water weight.

One effective way to hydrate is through fruits, vegetables, and herbs. According to Dr. Collins, the ultimate goal is to limit liquid intake to no more than 16 ounces per day. While this might seem extreme, if you consume truly hydrating foods, such as fruits, you won't need to drink as much liquid. Fruits contain what we call structured water.

We've previously discussed the existence of a fourth phase of water known as H3O2, which is structured water. The shapes of fruits are generally in platonic solid forms, allowing them to harness and enhance scalar frequencies from the sun. This structuring of liquid within fruits makes them exceptionally hydrating.

So, if you can aim to limit your liquid intake to no more than 16 ounces a day, that would be ideal. However, achieving this goal may take time and cannot be done overnight. Once your body adjusts, your kidneys will be better equipped to filter properly without becoming overwhelmed.

CHAPTER 72: POWER, LOVE, AND A SOUND MIND

2 Timothy 1:7 states, "For God hath not given us the spirit of fear; but of power, and of love, and of a sound mind (KJV)."

This verse highlights several important principles, particularly regarding the mind. While God does not give us a spirit of fear, we understand that fear comes from the adversary or opposition. The emotion and mindset of fear can negatively impact the kidney-bladder power line, which extends through various areas of the brain, including the cerebellum, occipital lobe, and the corpus callosum—crucial for communication between the left and right hemispheres.

Fear can inhibit the functioning of these brain regions, but God provides us with power. We know that true power comes through Jesus Christ. We gain this power through prayer, studying scripture, and making efforts to do good and keep God's commandments. Additionally, spending time outdoors in the sunlight also contributes to our sense of empowerment.

The verse also mentions love, which helps produce oxytocin—a hormone known to positively affect the brain. Furthermore, a sound mind is essential. As discussed in previous parts of this book, certain natural sounds and frequencies have healing properties. Sound entering one ear is processed by the opposite side of the brain, emphasizing the importance of auditory experiences for mental well-being.

These elements serve as tools provided by God to help us maintain a healthy mind. Therefore, the mention of a "sound mind" is significant.

We can also refer to James 1:8, which states that "a double minded man is unstable in all his ways (KJV)." The term "double minded" can have both spiritual and physical meanings. Spiritually, it implies the difficulty of serving both the Lord and opposing forces. Physically, it relates to the brain's dual hemispheres.

The left hemisphere of the brain is typically more analytical and mathematical, while the right hemisphere is more creative and artistic. When one side of the brain dominates, it can lead to instability, both mentally and physically. This imbalance may result in hypertonicity on one side of the body and hypotonicity (decreased muscle tone) on the other, creating further instability.

To promote better communication between the left and right hemispheres, it is essential to engage in activities that stimulate both sides of the brain. For instance, if you've engaged in a lot of spinning in one direction, it's important to spin in the opposite direction afterward. Balancing the brain also involves analytical tasks, such as math and science, alongside creative pursuits like art and music.

One of my favorite exercises for fostering left and right brain communication is juggling. There are numerous ways to achieve this balance, which I teach in the Healing Playbook membership. Ultimately, when your brain is balanced, your body will be also.

CHAPTER 73: MAKE STRAIGHT PATHS FOR YOUR FEET

In Hebrews 12:12-13, it states, "Wherefore lift up the hands which hang down, and the feeble knees; and make straight paths for your feet, lest that which is lame be turned out of the way; but let it rather be healed (KJV)." I love this scripture, especially the part about lifting up the hands that hang down.

This can refer to both our own hands and the hands of others. When we think of hands hanging down, we often picture someone who leans forward and feels defeated. We've talked about posture before, and lifting our hands can restore power and strength.

The passage also mentions feeble knees and encourages us to make straight paths for our feet. I often find that the feet are the foundation of the body. When the feet have issues, the rest of the body, particularly the knees, also suffer. This is increasingly common today due to modern footwear. Many modern shoes are narrow, which compresses the toes. Our toes are meant to spread out, and when they do, it not only enhances our balance and posture but also helps prevent ankle and knee injuries. It also activates nerves in our brain. As we discussed regarding the homunculus, a larger percentage of the nerves connected to the brain come from the face, hands, and feet.

One interesting principle I've learned is the benefit of wearing toe socks. They can help decrease or even eliminate snoring in some patients. I believe there is a neural connection between the toes and the throat.

To address this, consider wearing wider shoes for both casual and athletic purposes, and using toe socks that allow your toes to spread out. Additionally, there are exercises you can do to encourage space in the toes. One of my favorite tools for numerous patients is called toe spreaders—devices that you place between your toes to help them separate. This separation is similar to doing push-ups: if your hands are close together, it's harder due to decreased surface area. But when you spread your hands apart, you increase that area, making the push-up easier. The same principle applies to the toes; when they spread out, it's akin to performing a wider hand push-up, relieving pressure from the body all the way to the ankles, knees, hips, and back.

By providing your toes space, you'll notice improved posture, balance, and a reduction in injuries.

CHAPTER 74: DETAILED POWER LINES DESCRIPTIONS

In Revelation 1:14, the description of the Savior states that His head and hair were white like wool, as white as snow, and His eyes were like flames of fire (KJV). This powerful imagery carries significant meaning, particularly in terms of frequency and its underlying principles. The color white, which absorbs less negative energy, is noteworthy, and wool, which has a frequency of 5,000 Hertz according to Dr. Yellen (Crawford-Yellen, 2013). In my experience with patients, this is one of the frequencies that helps the vagus nerve for those in pain.

Additionally, snow, as previously mentioned, consists of organized water, showcasing a specific structure. The description of His eyes as flames of fire adds another layer of meaning. The color of fire often includes yellow, which resonates with the stomach power line, while those eyes connect neurologically to the occipital lobe of the brain—also linked to the bladder power line—and resonates with the color orange, which is commonly found in fire.

In Revelation 1:15, it states, "And his feet were like unto fine brass (KJV)." Brass tends to have a gold-like color, which again relates to yellow. The stomach power line extends down to the feet, reinforcing this yellow or brass association. The verse concludes with the statement that His voice was "as the sound of many waters (KJV)." Here, water is associated with the color blue, which resonates with the lung and large intestine power line, in which the voice is also connected to that power line.

All these descriptions of the Savior incorporate principles of frequency and physics, a fact that many people may not fully appreciate.

Another scripture that illustrates this concept of frequency in relation to the body is found in Revelation 10:1, which describes an angel with a rainbow upon his head (KJV). A rainbow is one way to visualize scalar frequencies, which are known to be healing for the body. My experience treating many patients suggests that one of the most effective locations for scalar frequency application is at the crown of the head. It also mentioned that the angel's face was like the sun. The sun, associated with yellow, resonates with the stomach power line, which passes through many facial muscles.

The angel's feet are also described as "pillars of fire (KJV)." Again, the stomach power line extends to the feet, and one of the colors associated with fire is orange, which resonates with kidney and bladder power lines, extending down to both the back and the soles of the feet.

These descriptions of various colors and their associated meanings—whether referring to the Savior or angels—are, in my opinion, divinely inspired. They use frequency and physics in ways that may not have been completely understood at the time. God possesses ultimate knowledge, and I believe these passages were crafted in the scriptures for a significant reason.

CHAPTER 75: COLD OR HOT

In Revelation 3:15, it states, "I know thy works, that thou art neither cold nor hot: I would thou wert cold or hot (KJV)." This passage pertains to a spiritual perspective; we cannot serve both God and the adversary. Ultimately, we can only serve God, but this also applies from a physical standpoint.

Today, our environment is often regulated by air conditioning and heating, so we rarely experience extreme temperatures. In contrast, our ancestors endured much more significant temperature variations. They faced prolonged periods of extreme heat and cold, which can be beneficial for our nervous systems. When our nervous systems are not challenged, they don't function optimally. This lack of challenge contributes to the prevalence of nervous system disorders in modern times.

One way to counteract this issue is to follow the scripture's guidance by embracing both hot and cold experiences. Let's start with cold. Cold showers or cold plunges are incredibly beneficial because they activate the vagus nerve through the trigeminal nerve (Richer et al., 2022). The vagus nerve stimulates the hypothalamus in the brain (Bonaz et al., 2017). The hypothalamus is vital for brain and body health. Additionally, I have seen that patients' exposure to cold water helps the lymphatic system drain, particularly the craniosacral pump, which is responsible for the lymphatic drainage of the brain.

Another advantage of cold exposure, such as cold plunges or showers, is that it enhances the body's ability to absorb ultraviolet light, which has healing properties.

Now, regarding heat, saunas come to mind. Research has documented the health benefits of sauna use, including weight loss (Laukkanen & Kunutsor, 2024).

The larger picture here is that both hot and cold therapies activate the spinothalamic tract (Al-Chalabi et al., 2023). This part of the nervous system plays a significant role in connecting the brain and body.

Instead of seeking comfort through moderate temperatures, consider incorporating both hot and cold therapies into your daily routine when possible. Doing so can lead to a healthier nervous system.

CHAPTER 76: GLASS, FIRE, AND HARPS

In Revelation 15:2, it describes those who have achieved victory over the beast, symbolizing victory over the adversary. This passage mentions a sea of glass mingled with fire, and the individuals stood on this sea of glass, holding the harps of God (KJV).

This imagery is intriguing because glass is made from silica, and quartz crystal is composed of silicon dioxide. Silica is known for its healing properties. When this material interacts with emitted frequencies, particularly light from fire, it enhances these frequencies. The mention of harps is significant as well; the vibrations and sounds produced by music can generate powerful frequencies from the glass, creating what is known as scalar frequency, which is healing for the body.

Overcoming opposition from the adversary involves both our spirit and our body, which together form our soul. An interesting aspect of harps is that they produce frequencies ranging from 31 Hertz to about 6,700 Hertz (Fox, 2024). This frequency range resonates with gamma waves in the brain, as well as all of the power lines of the organs, and parts of the vagus nerve. Therefore, these harmonies are beneficial for the body and promote healing.

It is fascinating to see another example of scalar frequency being emitted from the fire through the glass, as well as the sound of the harps reverberating through it.

CHAPTER 77: HIS NAME SHALL BE IN THEIR FOREHEADS

In Revelation 22:4, referring to the Savior, it says, "And they shall see his face," meaning the Saviors, and "his name shall be in their foreheads (KJV)."

There is another scripture that aligns with this theme, found in Revelation 14:1. It states, "And I looked, and lo, a Lamb stood on the mount Sion, and with him 144,000, having his Father's name written in their foreheads (KJV)." We know that the Lamb represents Jesus Christ.

What I love about this scripture, and the principle of frequency that applies to it, is that in ancient Ayurvedic medicine, one of the chakras, known as the third eye, is considered spiritual. The third eye is located just above the eyes, right at the forehead level. We see these two scriptures in the New Testament referring to having the Savior's name on our foreheads, indicating a spiritual principle.

Interestingly, the number 144,000 connects to the digital root of 3; when we break it down $(1 + 4 + 4 + 0 + 0 + 0)$, we see that $4 + 4 = 8$, and adding the 1 from 144,000 gives a total of 9. When we analyze the frequencies of numbers and the location of the forehead, which is associated with our spiritual center, we come to understand that ultimate healing comes from Jesus Christ. As I conclude this book, I hope you realize how important He is as the ultimate healer. Whenever we use frequency and physics to assist the body in healing, these are merely tools and instruments in His hands, and they all testify of Him.

Additionally, when referring to the forehead, consider that it is associated with the frontal lobe of the brain, which is responsible for learning new information. I hope that this book inspires you to read the scriptures more frequently. Throughout my experience treating thousands of patients with unique conditions, I have come to understand that the principles of frequency and physics permeate the scriptures. I hope you grasp this concept as well.

Importantly, when you have questions in life or need guidance from God, pray and ask your questions. You will find answers in the scriptures. This principle applies not only to the health of the body or spiritual matters, but also to your business, personal life, and relationships. Whenever you have righteous desires or goals, the answers can always be found in the scriptures. Reading and studying the scriptures engages the frontal lobe of the brain and is one of the ways the Lord communicates with us through the Spirit, also known as the Holy Ghost.

When we know something is true and inspired from above, we often feel peace, love, and happiness. One way I personally feel the Spirit is when I learn a new principle or seek Heavenly Father's guidance for health and come across a scripture that resonates with me. I think, "Oh, that makes sense!"—another manifestation of the Spirit.

I can promise you that if you strive to put the Lord first in your life, it will be the most effective way to achieve good health. This requires both faith and action. We express faith through prayer, and we demonstrate our commitment by reading the scriptures and implementing health principles discussed in this book. This includes consuming nutritious foods and spending time outdoors.

There are numerous principles we've learned together, and I am incredibly grateful for the knowledge the Lord has blessed us with in our time. We truly live in a special age as we prepare for His return. While none of us know exactly when He will come again, we do know He will. If we place our trust and faith in Him, He will help us overcome all challenges and enable us to thrive. The true Healing Playbook comes from our Savior, Jesus Christ, and through Him, there is no limit to healing.

ABOUT THE AUTHOR

Dr. Chase was born and raised in Dallas, Texas. At age 16 he became severely ill after a routine surgery that led him on a two year journey searching for answers. By the Grace of God, he was eventually introduced to the principles of frequency, physics, and nutrition. Using these principles he made a miraculous recovery, allowing him to graduate high school and attend Brigham Young University. He served a Spanish speaking Mission for the Church of Jesus Christ of Latter-Day Saints teaching the people of Mesa, Arizona the Gospel of Jesus Christ. Shortly after, he was married and sealed to his beautiful, and talented High School Sweetheart, Ashley, in the Dallas Texas Temple. He graduated from the University of Utah with a Bachelor's of Science in Health Promotion and Education and received a Diploma from the Institute for The Church of Jesus Christ of Latter-day Saints. Dr. Chase also graduated from Parker University as a Doctor of Chiropractic. He and his wife have four children; Reagan, Amanda, Collins, and Ox. Dr. Chase has worked alongside a variety of top medical practitioners and treated thousands of patients worldwide with some of the most unique conditions. Currently, Dr. Chase works alongside his wife, Ashley within their own business. Together, they co-founded Healing Playbook, LLC. Sharing Faith, Family, and Health content with people around the world through social media. You can find more information at

HealingPlaybook.com or follow them on Instagram @HealingPlaybook. As a Husband, Father, Author, Entrepreneur, and Inventor, Dr. Chase ultimately strives to teach people there is no limit to healing.

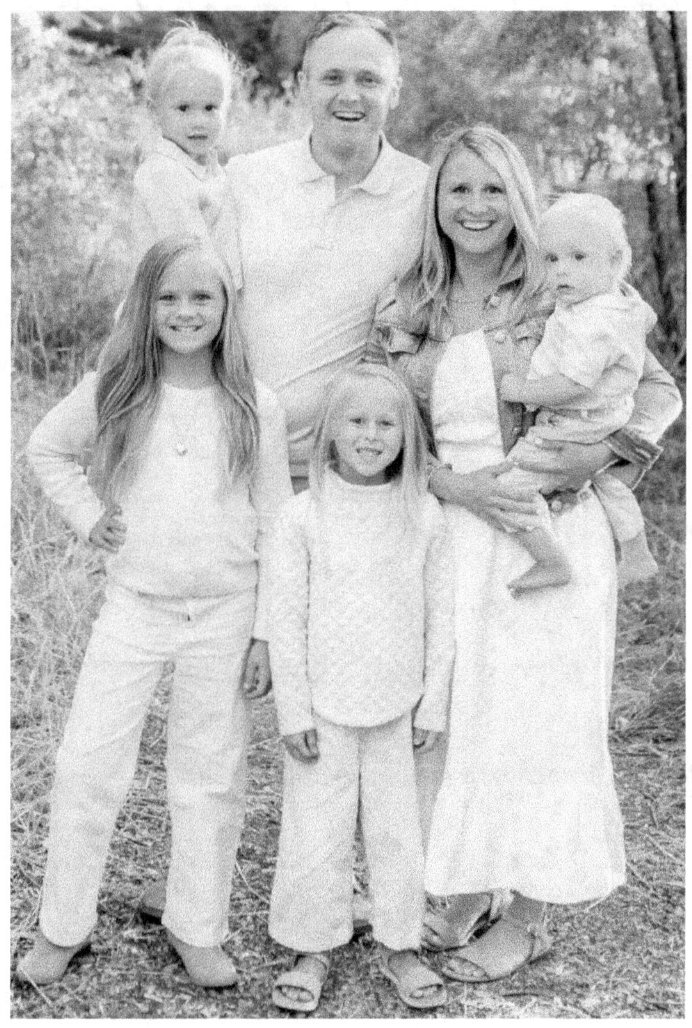

Sources Cited

Abegunawardana, S., Bodhika, J. A. P., Nanayakkara, S., Sonnadara, U., Fernando, M., & Cooray, V. (2014). Frequency Analysis of Thunder Features. *2014 International Conference on Lightning Protection (ICLP).*
https://www.researchgate.net/publication/309982045_Frequency_Analysis_of_Thunder_Features

Adaikkan, C., Middleton, S. J., Marco, A., Pao, P. C., Mathys, H., Kim, D. N., Gao, F., Young, J. Z., Suk, H. J., Boyden, E. S., McHugh, T. J., & Tsai, L. H. (2019). Gamma Entrainment Binds Higher-Order Brain Regions and Offers Neuroprotection. *Neuron, 102*(5), 929–943.e8. https://doi.org/10.1016/j.neuron.2019.04.011

Akimoto, K., Hu, A., Yamaguchi, T., & Kobayashi, H. (2018). Effect of 528 Hz music on the endocrine system and Autonomic Nervous System. *Health, 10*(09), 1159–1170. https://doi.org/10.4236/health.2018.109088

Al-Chalabi, M., Reddy, V., & Gupta, S. (2023). Neuroanatomy, Spinothalamic Tract. In *StatPearls.* StatPearls Publishing.

Bawankar, R., Singh, P., & Babu, S. (2014). Bioactive compounds and medicinal properties of aloe Vera L.: An update. *Journal of Plant*

Sciences (Science Publishing Group), *2*(3), 102. https://doi.org/10.11648/j.jps.20140203.11

Bedard, A. J. (2021). Waterfall low-frequency vibrations and infrasound: Implications for avian migration and hazard detection. *Journal of Comparative Physiology A*, *207*(6), 685–700. https://doi.org/10.1007/s00359-021-01510-5

Beko. (2018). *Old Olive trees in the Garden of Gethsemane, 12.jpg*. Wikimedia Commons. Wikimedia Commons. Retrieved 2025, from

https://commons.wikimedia.org/wiki/File:Old_Olive_trees_in_t he_Garden_of_Gethsemane,_12.jpg.

Boeckle, M., Preininger, D., & Hödl, W. (2009). Communication in noisy environments I: Acoustic signals of Staurois Latopalmatus Boulenger 1887. *Herpetologica*, *65*(2), 154–165. https://doi.org/10.1655/07-071r1.1

Bonaz, B., Sinniger, V., & Pellissier, S. (2017). The Vagus Nerve in the Neuro-Immune Axis: Implications in the Pathology of the Gastrointestinal Tract. *Frontiers in immunology*, *8*, 1452. https://doi.org/10.3389/fimmu.2017.01452

Butts, M., Sundaram, V. L., Murughiyan, U., Borthakur, A., & Singh, S. (2023). The Influence of Alcohol Consumption on Intestinal Nutrient Absorption: A Comprehensive Review. *Nutrients, 15*(7), 1571. https://doi.org/10.3390/nu15071571

Carr, A. C., & Maggini, S. (2017). Vitamin C and Immune Function. *Nutrients, 9*(11), 1211. https://doi.org/10.3390/nu9111211

Cate, C. T. (2004). Chapter 10 - Birdsong and evolution. In *Nature's Music: The Science of Birdsong* (pp. 296–317). essay, Academic Press. Retrieved 2025, from https://www.sciencedirect.com/topics/agricultural-and-biological-sciences/doves.

Crawford-Yellen, H. (2013, Winter). *Tikkun Olam to heal the world wearing healing flax-linen attire.* Academia.edu. https://www.academia.edu/39363092/Tikkun_Olam_to_Heal_the_World_Wearing_Healing_Flax_Linen_Attire

D'Alessandro, A., Nemkov, T., Sun, K., Liu, H., Song, A., Monte, A. A., Subudhi, A. W., Lovering, A. T., Dvorkin, D., Julian, C. G., Kevil, C. G., Kolluru, G. K., Shiva, S., Gladwin, M. T., Xia, Y., Hansen, K. C., & Roach, R. C. (2016). Altitudeomics: Red blood cell metabolic adaptation to high altitude hypoxia. *Journal of Proteome*

Research, *15*(10), 3883–3895. https://doi.org/10.1021/acs.jproteome.6b00733

Dimitrius. (2013). *Points of lung channel.* Wikimedia Commons. Wikimedia Commons. Retrieved February 4, 2023, from https://commons.wikimedia.org/wiki/File:Points_of_lung_chan nel_de.svg.

doTERRA. (2018). *Oil chemistry wheel.* doTERRA Oil Chemistry Wheel. https://media.doterra.com/us/en/flyers/doterra-oil-chemistry-wheel-2018.pdf

doTERRA. (2025, February 1). *Using the Wood Essential Oils.* doTERRA Essential Oils. https://www.doterra.com/US/en/blog/healthy-living-using-wood-oils

Elhefni, N., Ebada, S. S., Abdel-Aziz, M. M., Marwan, E. S. M., El-Sharkawy, S., & El-Neketi, M. (2023). Promising anti-*Helicobacter pylori* and anti-inflammatory metabolites from unused parts of *Phoenix dactylifera* CV 'Zaghloul': *in vitro* and *in silico* study. *Pharmaceutical Biology, 61*(1), 657–665. https://doi.org/10.1080/13880209.2023.2200841

Elmhalli, F., Garboui, S. S., Borg-Karlson, A.-K., Mozūraitis, R., Baldauf, S. L., & Grandi, G. (2019). The repellency and toxicity effects of essential oils from the Libyan plants Salvadora persica and rosmarinus officinalis against nymphs of Ixodes ricinus. *Experimental and Applied Acarology, 77*(4), 585–599. https://doi.org/10.1007/s10493-019-00373-5

Emoto, M. (2004). *The Hidden Messages in Water.* Beyond Words Pub.

Ferrari, S., Silva, M., Guarino, M., & Berckmans, D. (2008). Monitoring of swarming sounds in bee hives for early detection of the swarming period. *Computers and Electronics in Agriculture, 64*(1), 72–77. https://doi.org/10.1016/j.compag.2008.05.010

Fox, A. (2024, July 3). *Fundamental frequencies of musical notes in a=432 & A=440 hz.* My New Microphone. https://mynewmicrophone.com/fundamental-frequencies-of-musical-notes-in-a432-a440-hz/#Frequency-Range-Of-Concert-Harp

Harash, R. (2020, December 21). *Archaeologists recreate tiles of temple where jesus walked* . Reuters. https://www.reuters.com/article/world/middle-east/archaeologists-recreate-tiles-of-temple-where-jesus-walked-idUSKBN28V0X8/

Heij, C. J., & Verboom, W. C. (2021). Bird vocalizations: chirps of a male House sparrow (Passer domesticus). *JunoBioacoustics*, 1–6.

https://www.researchgate.net/publication/351287282_Bird_voca lizations_chirps_of_a_male_House_sparrow_Passer_domesticus

Kéver, L., Colleye, O., Lugli, M., Lecchini, D., Lerouvreur, F., Herrel, A., & Parmentier, E. (2014). Sound production in onuxodon fowleri (carapidae) and its amplification by the host shell. *Journal of Experimental Biology*, *217*(24), 4283–4294. https://doi.org/10.1242/jeb.109363

Khan, S. U., Jannat, S., Shaukat, H., Unab, S., Tanzeela, Akram, M., Khan Khattak, M. N., Soto, M. V., Khan, M. F., Ali, A., & Rizvi, S. S. R. (2023). Stress Induced Cortisol Release Depresses The Secretion of Testosterone in Patients With Type 2 Diabetes Mellitus. *Clinical medicine insights. Endocrinology and diabetes*, *16*, 11795514221145841. https://doi.org/10.1177/11795514221145841

King James Bible (KJV). (2013). The Church of Jesus Christ of Latter-day Saints. https://www.churchofjesuschrist.org/study/scriptures/nt?lang=e ng 99

Kurotchenko, S. P., Subbotina, T. I., Tuktamyshev, I. I., Tuktamyshev, I. S.h, Khadartsev, A. A., & Yashin, A. A. (2003). Shielding effect of mineral schungite during electromagnetic irradiation of rats. *Bulletin of experimental biology and medicine, 136*(5), 458–459. https://doi.org/10.1023/b:bebm.0000017092.52535.f8

Kutsch, W. (1973). The influence of age and culture-temperature on the wing-beat frequency of the Migratory Locust, Locusta Migratoria. *Journal of Insect Physiology, 19*(4), 763–772. https://doi.org/10.1016/0022-1910(73)90148-0

Laukkanen, J. A., & Kunutsor, S. K. (2024). The multifaceted benefits of passive heat therapies for extending the healthspan: A comprehensive review with a focus on Finnish sauna. *Temperature (Austin, Tex.), 11*(1), 27–51. https://doi.org/10.1080/23328940.2023.2300623

Lass, J. (2021). *Snowflake (lumehelves).* Wikimedia Commons. Wikimedia Commons. Retrieved 2025, from https://commons.wikimedia.org/wiki/File:Snowflake_(lumehelves).jpg.

Leidus, I. (2022). *Fig (Ficus carica) fruit halved.* Wikimedia Commons. Wikimedia Commons. Retrieved 2025, from https://commons.wikimedia.org/wiki/File:Fig_(Ficus_carica)_fruit_halved.jpg.

Lombardo, M., Vigezzi, A., Ietto, G., Franchi, C., Iori, V., Masci, F., Scorza, A., Macchi, S., Iovino, D., Parise, C., & Carcano, G. (2021). Role of vitamin D serum levels in prevention of primary and recurrent melanoma. *Scientific Reports*, *11*(1). https://doi.org/10.1038/s41598-021-85294-3

Mads00. (2016). *Neural pathway diagram.svg*. Wikimedia Commons. Wikimedia Commons. Retrieved November 21, 2024, from https://commons.wikimedia.org/wiki/File:Neural_pathway_diag ram.svg.

Martorell, A. J., Paulson, A. L., Suk, H. J., Abdurrob, F., Drummond, G. T., Guan, W., Young, J. Z., Kim, D. N., Kritskiy, O., Barker, S. J., Mangena, V., Prince, S. M., Brown, E. N., Chung, K., Boyden, E. S., Singer, A. C., & Tsai, L. H. (2019). Multi-sensory Gamma Stimulation Ameliorates Alzheimer's-Associated Pathology and Improves Cognition. *Cell*, *177*(2), 256–271.e22. https://doi.org/10.1016/j.cell.2019.02.014

Mawa, S., Husain, K., & Jantan, I. (2013). Ficus carica L. (Moraceae): Phytochemistry, Traditional Uses and Biological Activities. Evidence-based complementary and alternative medicine : eCAM, 2013, 974256. https://doi.org/10.1155/2013/974256

Mehridinov, H. (2023). *Honey locust (Gleditsia triacanthos) branches.* Wikimedia Commons. Wikimedia Commons. Retrieved 2025, from

https://commons.wikimedia.org/wiki/File:Honey_locust_(Gledit sia_tiacanthos)_branches.jpg.

Mosher, R. (2022, April). *Silver: Metal of Many Faces.* Dartmouth Toxic Metals. https://sites.dartmouth.edu/toxmetal/more-metals/silver-metal-of-many-faces/#:~:text=The%20Greeks%20and%20Romans%20stored,w as%20claiming%20their%20neighbors'%20lives.

Mukherjee, T. (2024). *Oriental turtle dove by Tisha Mukherjee 02.jpg.* Wikimedia Commons. Wikimedia Commons. Retrieved 2025, from

https://commons.wikimedia.org/wiki/File:Oriental_turtle_dove_ by_Tisha_Mukherjee_02.jpg.

Pollack, G. (n.d.). *Research.* pollacklab. https://www.pollacklab.org/research#:~:text=The%20Pollack% 20laboratory%20centers%20largely,in%20health%2C%20includin g%20cell%20biology.

Ramey, D., & Buell, P. D. (2004). A true history of acupuncture. *Focus on Alternative and Complementary Therapies*, *9*(4), 269–273. https://doi.org/10.1211/fact.2004.00244

Richer, R., Zenkner, J., Küderle, A., Rohleder, N., & Eskofier, B. M. (2022). Vagus activation by Cold Face Test reduces acute psychosocial stress responses. *Scientific reports*, *12*(1), 19270. https://doi.org/10.1038/s41598-022-23222-9

Rowan. (2007). *Inside the crypta of Deendera, Egypt.* Wikimedia Commons. Photograph, Dendera; Wikimedia Commons. Retrieved January 11, 2025, from https://commons.wikimedia.org/wiki/File:Dendera03.jpg.

Suk, H.-J., Buie, N., Xu, G., Banerjee, A., Boyden, E. S., & Tsai, L.-H. (2023). Vibrotactile stimulation at gamma frequency mitigates pathology related to neurodegeneration and improves motor function. *Frontiers in Aging Neuroscience*, *15*. https://doi.org/10.3389/fnagi.2023.1129510

Szameitat, D. P., Darwin, C. J., Szameitat, A. J., Wildgruber, D., & Alter, K. (2011). Formant characteristics of human laughter. *Journal of Voice*, *25*(1), 32–37. https://doi.org/10.1016/j.jvoice.2009.06.010

Tang, J. Y., Yeh, T. W., Huang, Y. T., Wang, M. H., & Jang, L. S. (2019). Effects of extremely low-frequency electromagnetic fields on B16F10 cancer cells. *Electromagnetic biology and medicine*, *38*(2), 149–157. https://doi.org/10.1080/15368378.2019.1591438

Teixeira, J. A. (2024, October 5). *Bonded to jesus christ: Becoming the salt of the Earth*. Homepage - The Church of Jesus Christ of Latter-day Saints. https://www.churchofjesuschrist.org/study/general-conference/2024/10/22teixeira?lang=eng

Torres, R., Koutakis, P., & Forsse, J. (2021). The effects of different exercise intensities and modalities on cortisol production in healthy individuals: A Review. *Journal of Exercise and Nutrition*, *4*(4). https://doi.org/10.53520/jen2021.103108

Uddin, I., & Kanatas, A. (2014). Oral health: Salvadora Persica. *British Dental Journal*, *216*(3), 98–98. https://doi.org/10.1038/sj.bdj.2014.53

Vila Domínguez, A., Ayerbe Algaba, R., Miró Canturri, A., Rodríguez Villodres, Á., & Smani, Y. (2020). Antibacterial Activity of Colloidal Silver against Gram-Negative and Gram-Positive Bacteria. *Antibiotics (Basel, Switzerland)*, *9*(1), 36. https://doi.org/10.3390/antibiotics9010036

Wang, C., Bókkon, I., Dai, J., & Antal, I. (2011). Spontaneous and visible light-induced ultraweak photon emission from Rat eyes.

Brain Research, 1369, 1–9. https://doi.org/10.1016/j.brainres.2010.10.077

Zielińska, A., Wójcicki, K., Klensporf-Pawlik, D., Dias-Ferreira, J., Lucarini, M., Durazzo, A., Lucariello, G., Capasso, R., Santini, A., Souto, E. B., Nowak, I., & Cuisset, A. (2020). Chemical and physical properties of meadowfoam seed oil and extra virgin olive oil: Focus on vibrational spectroscopy. *Journal of Spectroscopy, 2020,* 1–9. https://doi.org/10.1155/2020/8870170

Zuo, Y., Li, Y., Gu, X., & Lei, Z. (2021). The correlation between selenium levels and autoimmune thyroid disease: A systematic review and meta-analysis. *Annals of Palliative Medicine, 10*(4), 4398–4408. https://doi.org/10.21037/apm-21-449

Index

U

UV light, 102

V

Vagus nerve, 171, 172, 173, 174, 175, 186, 187, 220, 223, 225
Vinegar, 186
Vitamin C, 26, 234

W

Weightlifting, 59
Wilderness, 64, 65, 66, 71, 104
World war II, 96

Y

Yoga, 112

Z

Zacharia, 20